GRAVE'S DISEASE COOKBOOK FOR BEGINNERS

50 Super Easy, Delicious Recipe and a 28-Day Meal Plan to Calm Your Thyroid, Reduce Flares, and Reclaim Your Energy

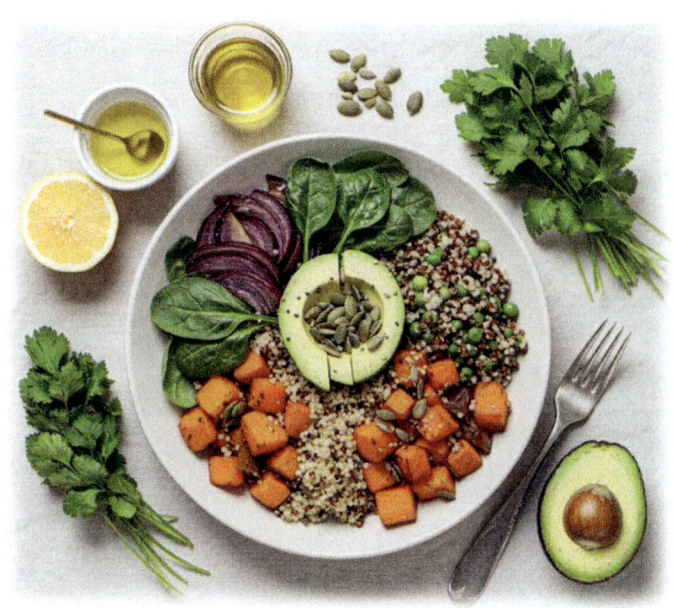

Thalia Rowen

Copyright © 2025 by Thalia Rowen

All rights reserved.

No part of this publication may be reproduced, stored in a retrieval system, or transmitted in any form or by any means—electronic, mechanical, photocopying, recording, or otherwise—without prior written permission from the publisher, except in the case of brief quotations embodied in critical articles or reviews.

This book is intended for informational purposes only. It is not a substitute for professional medical advice, diagnosis, or treatment. Always seek the advice of your physician or other qualified healthcare provider before starting any diet or health program.

Names, characters, and recipes in this book are original or adapted for educational purposes. Any resemblance to actual persons, living or dead, is purely coincidental.

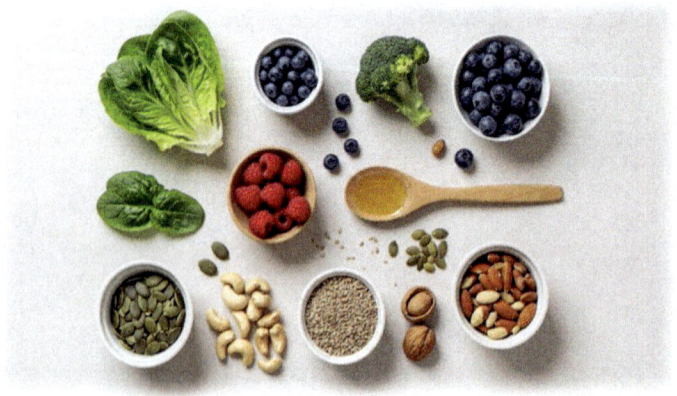

Gratitude

Writing this book has been one of the most rewarding and transformative journeys of my life, and I am deeply grateful to everyone who made it possible.

To my readers, thank you for trusting me to walk alongside you on your healing journey. Whether you were recently diagnosed with Graves' disease or are simply seeking a better way to nourish your body, I am honored to be part of your path toward balance and wellness. Your courage to take control of your health is inspiring, and I hope this book brings you clarity, comfort, and confidence in your daily choices.

This cookbook belongs to:

_____

_____

_____

_____

_____

_____

TABLE OF CONTENT

INTRODUCTION 1

CHAPTER 1: 3

UNDERSTANDING GRAVES' DISEASE AND YOUR THYROID 3

    What Is Graves' Disease? 3

    The Role of The Thyroid in Your Body 4

    Common Symptoms and Challenges 5

    How Diet Impacts Thyroid Function 6

    Your Journey to Symptom Management 7

CHAPTER 2: 9

THE NUTRITION-THYROID CONNECTION 9

    Foods That Support Thyroid Health 9

    Foods To Minimize or Avoid 13

    Balancing Your Plate for Optimal Thyroid Function 17

CHAPTER 3: 21

KITCHEN ESSENTIALS AND MEAL PREP 21

    Stocking Your Pantry for Success 21

    Time-Saving Meal Preparation Techniques 24

    Essential Cooking Equipment 26

    Reading Labels and Shopping Smart 27

    Managing Food Sensitivities 29

CHAPTER 4: 33

YOUR 28-DAY MEAL PLAN FOR THYROID HEALING 33

    Week 1: Shopping List 33

Week 1: Meal Prep Guidelines 35

Week 1: Meal Plan 36

Week 2: Building Consistency and Balance 40

Week 2: Shopping List 40

Week 2: Meal Prep Guidelines 42

Week 2: Meal Plan 43

WEEK 3: DEEPENING THE HEALING PROCESS 46

Week 3: Shopping List 46

Week 3: Meal Prep Guidelines 48

Week 3: Meal Plan 49

Week 4: Sustaining Your Progress for Long-Term Health ... 52

Week 4: Shopping List 52

Week 4: Meal Prep Guidelines 54

Week 4: Meal Plan 55

BREAKFAST RECIPES 59

MAIN DISHES 76

SIDES, SALADS, AND SOUPS 108

SNACKS AND DESSERTS 125

BONUS 149

CONCLUSION 165

ABOUT THE AUTHOR 167

BONUS INSIDE!

Healing Smoothie Recipes to Nourish Your Thyroid Naturally

Because you're here, I've got something extra just for you—and it's already included in this book.

At the very end of your 28-day journey, you'll unlock a special bonus section packed with 10+ thyroid-friendly smoothie recipes designed to support healing, reduce flares, and boost your energy.

Why Smoothies?

When dealing with Graves' Disease, there are days when cooking feels like too much. That's where smoothies shine—they're quick, calming, and loaded with the nutrients your body is craving.

- Inside the bonus section, you'll find:

- Easy-to-make, nutrient-rich smoothies

- Soothing blends for flare-up days

- Energizing options to kickstart your morning

- Naturally delicious, without triggering ingredients

These recipes are a powerful companion to your meal plan—perfect for days when you need a gentle, healing reset.

So, as you flip through this book, know there's a bonus waiting for you at the finish line—because your health journey deserves a delicious reward.

With care,

Thalia Rowen

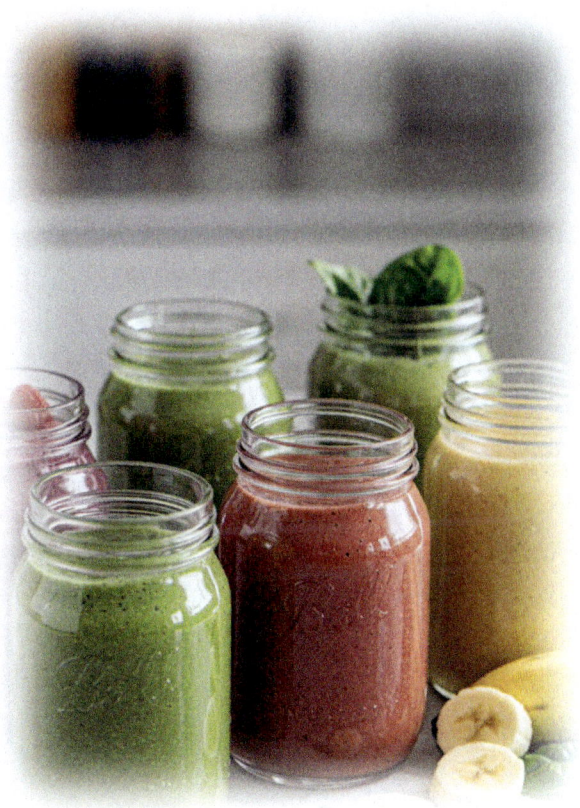

INTRODUCTION

Did you know that Graves' disease affects roughly 1 in every 200 people, with women being up to ten times more likely to develop it than men? When I first heard that statistic, I felt like just another number—one more person in a sea of many, struggling to understand what was happening to my body.

Before I was diagnosed, I knew something was off. My heart raced even when I was sitting still. I was losing weight without trying, felt anxious for no reason, and my hands trembled like I had too much coffee—except I hadn't had any. At first, I brushed it off, thinking it was just stress or maybe burnout. But when my eyes started feeling dry and irritated and I couldn't sleep through the night anymore, I knew I had to see a doctor.

Hearing the words "Graves' disease" was both a relief and a shock. On one hand, I finally had a name for what was happening. On the other hand, I was overwhelmed with questions: What does this mean for my future? Will I ever feel normal again? What can I do to help my body heal?

One of the biggest shifts I made—and one that truly changed everything—was adjusting the way I eat. At first, it felt like a minefield. Some foods made my symptoms worse. Others seemed to help calm the storm inside me. I was desperate for guidance, but so much of the information out there was conflicting, confusing, or just plain hard to follow.

That's why I created this cookbook.

I wanted something that was actually helpful—not just a list of dos and don'ts, but a guide you can turn to every day. Whether you're newly diagnosed or simply trying to regain control of your health, I've been there. I know what it feels like to stare at your plate wondering if your next bite is helping or hurting you.

This book is filled with recipes that are not only thyroid-friendly, but also nourishing, simple, and delicious. More than that, it's built around understanding the connection between nutrition and thyroid health—because food can be powerful medicine when used the right way.

And listen, you don't need to be a gourmet chef or have a fancy kitchen to start feeling better. You just need some clear guidance, a little inspiration, and the willingness to try.

So, here's my invitation to you: Take this journey with me. Explore what it feels like to eat in a way that supports your body, calms your symptoms, and empowers you every day. You deserve to feel good again—and I truly believe this is a step in the right direction.

CHAPTER 1:

UNDERSTANDING GRAVES' DISEASE AND YOUR THYROID

When you're first diagnosed with Graves' disease, it can feel like your body has turned against you—and you have no idea how to get back in control. Your heart is racing, your emotions are on a rollercoaster, and you're constantly fatigued despite getting enough sleep. The symptoms can be overwhelming, but understanding what's happening inside your body is the first powerful step toward healing.

What Is Graves' Disease?

Graves' disease is an autoimmune disorder, which means your immune system—the very thing designed to protect you—is mistakenly attacking your thyroid gland. The result? Your thyroid begins to work overtime, producing excess thyroid hormones in a condition called hyperthyroidism.

What makes Graves' disease unique is that it's the most common cause of hyperthyroidism and often comes with specific symptoms like bulging eyes (a condition called

Graves' ophthalmopathy), anxiety, weight loss, and heat intolerance. It's not something you "catch," and it's definitely not your fault. Genetics, stress, and even environmental triggers can all play a role in its development.

But while you can't turn off your immune system's response with the flick of a switch, there are things you can do to support your body—starting with understanding the thyroid itself.

The Role of The Thyroid in Your Body

Your thyroid is a butterfly-shaped gland located at the base of your neck. Despite its small size, it has a massive impact on nearly every system in your body. It produces hormones—primarily T3 (triiodothyronine) and T4 (thyroxine)—that regulate your metabolism, energy levels, heart rate, temperature, and even mood.

When the thyroid is functioning properly, you likely don't think twice about it. But when it's overactive, as it is in Graves' disease, it can feel like your body is constantly on fast-forward. It's like your internal thermostat is broken, and everything—your heart, digestion, nervous system—is racing to keep up.

This is why symptom management becomes so crucial. You're not just dealing with one issue; you're managing a complex cascade of effects that all start with the thyroid.

Common Symptoms and Challenges

Graves' disease manifests differently for everyone, but there are a few common threads:

- Unexplained weight loss
- Rapid or irregular heartbeat
- Anxiety, irritability, and mood swings
- Tremors in the hands and fingers
- Heat sensitivity and excessive sweating
- Fatigue and muscle weakness
- Sleep disturbances
- Bulging eyes or eye discomfort
- Menstrual irregularities

It's not just the physical symptoms that take a toll—it's the emotional and mental load too. You may feel like you're losing control of your own body. Social outings might become draining. Simple tasks may feel monumental. And worst of all, some people might not understand what you're going through because on the outside, you look fine.

But here's the truth: your experience is valid, and you're not alone.

How Diet Impacts Thyroid Function

While there's no "magic food" that can cure Graves' disease, what you eat plays a major role in how you feel each day. Certain foods can either support your thyroid or aggravate your symptoms. For example, too much iodine can over-stimulate the thyroid, while selenium and zinc can help regulate hormone production and reduce inflammation.

A balanced, anti-inflammatory diet can also help stabilize energy levels, improve digestion, and support your immune system—essential when you're living with an autoimmune condition. The key is to fuel your body with nutrient-rich, whole foods that promote healing rather than create more stress.

And remember, food isn't just fuel—it's information. The right nutrients can signal to your body that it's safe, calm, and supported. That's powerful.

Your Journey to Symptom Management

Managing Graves' disease isn't about perfection. It's about learning to tune in to your body, recognize what helps and what doesn't, and making choices that bring you closer to balance.

That's where this cookbook comes in. My goal is to give you the tools and confidence to use food as part of your healing plan. Whether you're newly diagnosed or looking to gain more control over your symptoms, you'll find recipes and insights throughout this book to help you feel more grounded, nourished, and empowered.

Let's dive deeper, together.

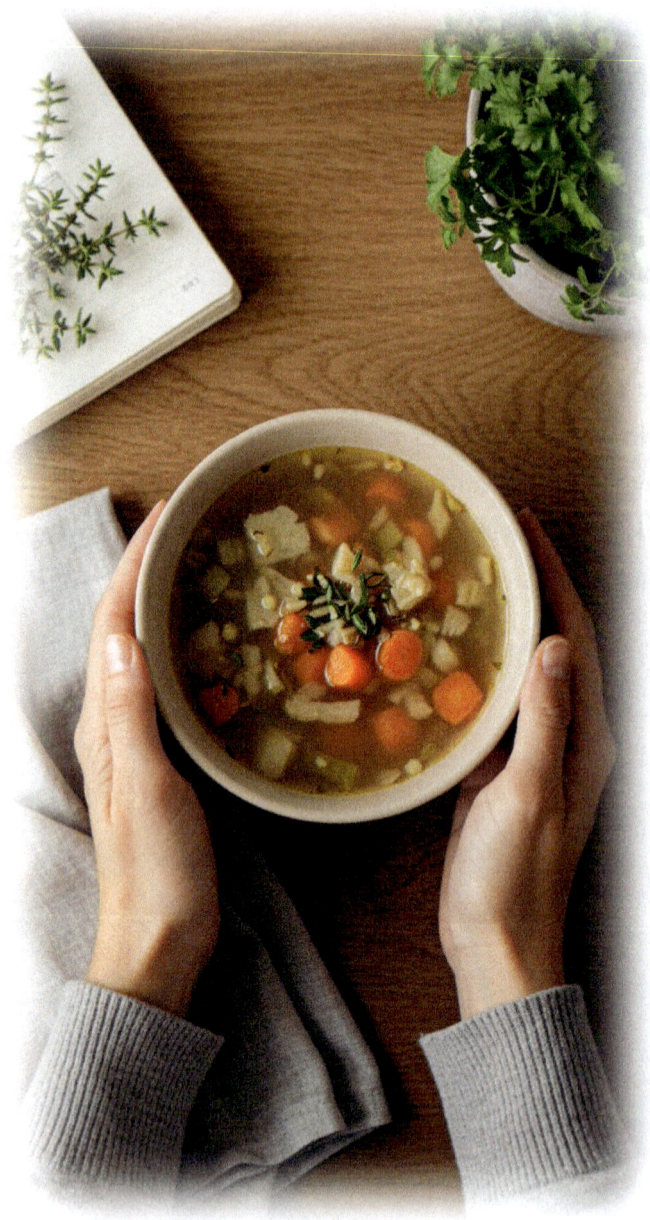

CHAPTER 2:

THE NUTRITION-THYROID CONNECTION

When living with Graves' disease, one of the most powerful tools you have at your disposal is your fork. What you eat on a daily basis can significantly influence how you feel, how well your thyroid functions, and how effectively you manage symptoms. Nutrition won't cure Graves' disease, but it can absolutely support your healing and improve your quality of life.

In this chapter, we'll explore the foods that nourish and protect your thyroid, the ones that may work against it, and how to create balanced meals that truly support your journey back to wellness.

Foods That Support Thyroid Health

The right foods can help reduce inflammation, support your immune system, replenish vital nutrients, and regulate hormone production. Here are some of the most important nutrients and food groups to prioritize:

Selenium-Rich Foods

Selenium is a trace mineral that plays a critical role in thyroid hormone metabolism and immune function. It helps convert the thyroid hormone T4 into its active form, T3, and also acts as a powerful antioxidant, helping to reduce inflammation and oxidative stress in the thyroid gland.

Best sources:

- Brazil nuts (just 1-2 per day can provide your full daily selenium needs)
- Sardines and tuna
- Eggs
- Sunflower seeds
- Shiitake mushrooms

Tip: Be cautious not to overdo it—selenium is essential, but too much can be harmful. Moderation is key.

Zinc Sources

Zinc is another mineral that supports thyroid hormone production and helps regulate immune responses. People with Graves' disease may be at risk for zinc deficiency due to inflammation and increased metabolic demands.

Best sources:

- Oysters (one of the richest sources)
- Beef and lamb
- Pumpkin seeds
- Chickpeas
- Cashews

Adding zinc-rich foods regularly can help maintain thyroid hormone levels and keep immune function in check.

Antioxidant-Rich Fruits and Vegetables

Chronic inflammation is a major factor in autoimmune diseases like Graves'. Antioxidants help fight free radicals that can damage thyroid tissue and exacerbate symptoms.

Best options include:

- Berries (blueberries, strawberries, raspberries)
- Leafy greens (spinach, kale, Swiss chard)
- Cruciferous vegetables (broccoli, cauliflower—lightly cooked to reduce goitrogens)
- Carrots and sweet potatoes (rich in beta-carotene)
- Red cabbage and beets

Try to "eat the rainbow" every day—colorful produce provides a wide range of antioxidants and phytonutrients to support healing.

Healthy Fats

Anti-inflammatory fats are essential for hormone production, brain health, and reducing inflammation in the body. They also help you absorb fat-soluble vitamins (A, D, E, K), which are vital for thyroid function.

Great sources include:

- Avocados
- Extra virgin olive oil
- Fatty fish like salmon, sardines, and mackerel
- Chia seeds and flaxseeds
- Walnuts

Avoid trans fats and heavily processed oils—these can worsen inflammation and interfere with hormonal balance.

Quality Proteins

Your body needs protein to repair tissues, regulate immune function, and produce thyroid hormones. A

Graves'-related high metabolism may increase your body's protein demands, so ensuring adequate intake is essential.

Excellent options include:

- Pasture-raised poultry
- Wild-caught fish
- Eggs
- Lentils and legumes
- Quinoa and tofu (in moderation, more on soy later)
- Bone broth (rich in collagen and minerals)

Protein helps keep you full, stabilizes blood sugar, and supports muscle health—especially important when dealing with fatigue and muscle weakness.

Foods To Minimize or Avoid

Just as some foods support thyroid health, others can hinder it—especially when consumed frequently. For people with Graves' disease, certain foods can trigger immune responses, disrupt hormone levels, or increase inflammation. While everyone's body is different, these are the most common culprits to be mindful of.

Highly Processed Foods

Processed foods are often high in unhealthy fats, sugar, additives, and preservatives, all of which can cause inflammation and strain your immune system. They may also be low in the nutrients your body desperately needs.

Examples include:

- Packaged snacks (chips, crackers, cookies)
- Fast food
- Frozen meals with long ingredient lists
- Artificial sweeteners and flavorings
- Aim to choose whole, minimally processed foods whenever possible.

Excessive Iodine Sources

Iodine is essential for thyroid function, but too much—especially in Graves' disease can worsen hyperthyroidism. While iodine deficiency is linked to hypothyroidism, excessive intake can trigger or exacerbate autoimmune activity in Graves'.

Foods high in iodine to limit or avoid:

- Iodized salt (consider using unrefined sea salt in moderation)
- Kelp and seaweed

- Iodine supplements (unless prescribed by your doctor)
- Talk with your healthcare provider before adding any iodine-rich foods or supplements to your diet.

Gluten (for Sensitive Individuals)

There's a known link between autoimmune thyroid conditions and gluten sensitivity. Some individuals with Graves' disease may have or develop celiac disease, or experience heightened inflammation due to gluten exposure.

If you suspect sensitivity, consider avoiding:

- Wheat, barley, rye
- Conventional breads, pastas, and baked goods
- Try gluten-free whole grains like brown rice, quinoa, buckwheat, and certified gluten-free oats instead.

Soy Products

Soy contains compounds called isoflavones that may interfere with thyroid hormone absorption, especially in high amounts. While occasional consumption may be fine for many, those with active Graves' symptoms may benefit from limiting soy intake.

Foods to minimize:

- Soy milk
- Tofu and tempeh
- Soy protein powders
- Edamame
- Processed vegetarian meat substitutes

If you choose to eat soy, opt for fermented varieties (like tempeh or miso) and consume in moderation.

Caffeine and Alcohol

Both caffeine and alcohol can stimulate the nervous system, exacerbate anxiety, and interfere with sleep—all things that people with Graves' disease often struggle with already. They may also interfere with medication absorption and liver function.

Try to limit or avoid:

- Coffee and energy drinks
- Black and green tea (caffeinated versions)
- Alcoholic beverages

Consider herbal teas, decaf coffee, or chicory root beverages as gentler alternatives.

High-Sugar Foods

Sugar causes inflammation, disrupts blood sugar levels, and can exacerbate fatigue and brain fog. It also feeds gut dysbiosis, which is increasingly linked to autoimmune flare-ups.

Minimize foods like:

- Soda and sweetened beverages
- Candy and sweets
- Baked goods made with refined sugar
- Sweetened cereals

Natural alternatives like fruit, raw honey (in moderation), or dates can satisfy your sweet tooth without sending your system into overdrive.

Balancing Your Plate for Optimal Thyroid Function

Now that you know what to focus on and what to avoid, the next step is learning how to build a balanced plate that supports your thyroid every single day.

Here's a simple visual guide you can follow for every meal:

1. Start with a Quality Protein (¼ of your plate)

Protein stabilizes energy, keeps you full, and supports muscle and immune health. Choose lean meats, eggs, legumes, or fish.

2. Add Non-Starchy Veggies (½ of your plate)

Go big on the greens, carrots, broccoli, bell peppers, and cruciferous veggies (lightly cooked). These are your antioxidant powerhouses.

3. Include Healthy Fats (a thumb-sized amount or drizzle)

Add olive oil, avocado slices, nuts, or seeds to help with hormone absorption and fight inflammation.

4. Choose Complex Carbohydrates (¼ of your plate)

Opt for quinoa, sweet potatoes, brown rice, or gluten-free oats. These provide lasting energy without blood sugar crashes.

5. Hydrate and Stay Mindful

Drink water throughout the day. Herbal teas can also help with digestion and relaxation. Mindful eating—slowing down and chewing thoroughly—helps you tune in to your body's needs.

Your plate is more than just food—it's part of your medicine cabinet. By choosing ingredients that work with your body rather than against it, you give yourself the power to manage Graves' disease from the inside out.

In the next chapter, we'll dive into pantry essentials and meal planning to make eating this way realistic, affordable, and enjoyable. You don't have to overhaul everything at once—but each smart choice adds up.

You're learning to nourish your body with purpose. And that's a beautiful step toward healing

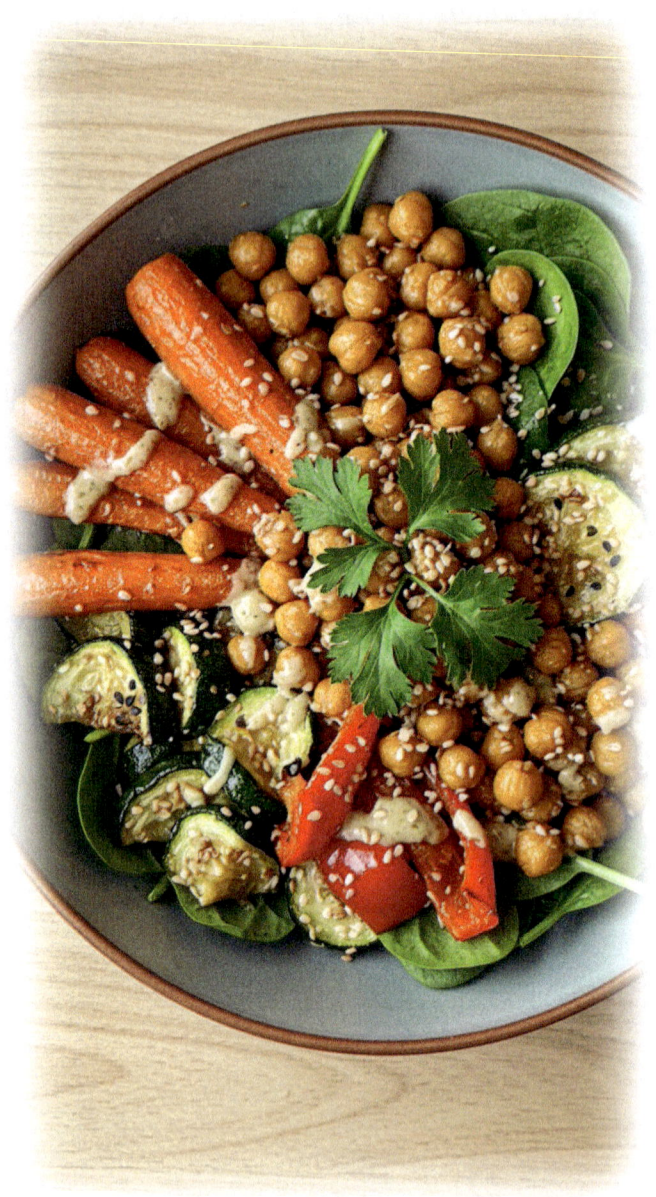

CHAPTER 3:

KITCHEN ESSENTIALS AND MEAL PREP

Starting a new way of eating can feel intimidating—especially when you're managing symptoms like fatigue, brain fog, or anxiety from Graves' disease. But having the right tools, ingredients, and habits in place can make a world of difference. Think of your kitchen as your wellness sanctuary, and setting it up well is the first step toward taking back control of your health.

This chapter will guide you through building a thyroid-friendly pantry, meal prepping with confidence, cooking with ease, shopping smarter, and navigating food sensitivities.

Stocking Your Pantry for Success

Your pantry is the foundation of your healing meals. A well-stocked pantry saves you time, reduces stress, and keeps you consistent in making thyroid-supportive choices.

Here's what to focus on:

Whole Grains (Gluten-Free or Low-Gluten)

- Brown rice
- Quinoa
- Buckwheat
- Millet
- Certified gluten-free oats
- Amaranth

Why it matters: These grains are rich in fiber and B vitamins, which support digestion, energy, and hormone regulation—without triggering potential gluten sensitivities.

Legumes & Plant-Based Proteins

- Lentils (red, green, black)
- Chickpeas
- Black beans
- Split peas

Note: If you have digestive sensitivities, start with small portions and soak or cook thoroughly to aid digestion.

Healthy Fats & Oils

- Extra virgin olive oil

- Avocado oil
- Coconut oil (for high-heat cooking)
- Raw nuts and seeds (almonds, walnuts, pumpkin seeds, chia seeds, flaxseeds)
- Nut butters (unsweetened almond or cashew butter)

Why it matters: These fats reduce inflammation and support hormone production.

Canned & Jarred Goods

- Wild-caught canned salmon or sardines (rich in omega-3s and selenium)
- No-sugar-added tomato paste or crushed tomatoes
- Full-fat coconut milk (for creamy sauces and soups)
- Bone broth or vegetable broth (for gut support and minerals)

Herbs, Spices & Condiments

- Turmeric, ginger, cinnamon, cumin, rosemary, and thyme (anti-inflammatory and antioxidant-rich)
- Apple cider vinegar

- Tamari or coconut aminos (soy sauce alternatives)
- Himalayan pink salt or sea salt (use in moderation)

Avoid: Conventional soy sauce, MSG, and condiments with added sugar or artificial ingredients.

Sweeteners (Used Sparingly)

- Raw honey (local, if possible)
- Maple syrup
- Medjool dates

These natural sweeteners offer antioxidants and are less likely to spike blood sugar when used in moderation.

Time-Saving Meal Preparation Techniques

When fatigue or brain fog hits, the last thing you want to do is cook from scratch every single meal. That's why meal prep is your secret weapon—it reduces decision fatigue, ensures healthy choices are ready when you need them, and gives you back time and energy.

Batch Cooking

- Set aside a couple of hours once or twice a week to batch cook:
- Proteins (grilled chicken, baked salmon, lentil patties)
- Roasted vegetables (sweet potatoes, carrots, cauliflower)
- Grains (quinoa, rice, gluten-free pasta)
- Soups or stews (freeze in single-serve portions)
- Use airtight containers to keep things fresh and organized.

Prep Ingredients, Not Just Meals

- Wash and chop produce in advance
- Pre-portion snacks (nuts, fruits, hummus with veggies)
- Make salad dressings and sauces ahead of time
- This makes assembling meals quick and easy—even on your busiest or lowest-energy days.

Use the "Cook Once, Eat Twice" Strategy

Make enough at dinner to turn into lunch the next day. For example:

- Roast chicken → chicken and veggie stir-fry
- Lentil soup → thinned with broth for a next-day stew
- Quinoa bowl → turned into a salad with greens and avocado

Embrace Freezer-Friendly Recipes

Soups, stews, meatballs, and energy bites all freeze well and reheat beautifully—ideal for days when cooking feels impossible.

Essential Cooking Equipment

You don't need a gourmet kitchen to cook healing meals, but a few reliable tools can make a huge difference in your efficiency and enjoyment.

Must-Have Essentials

1. High-Quality Knife & Cutting Board: For chopping fruits, vegetables, and proteins with ease.
2. Large Baking Sheet: For roasting vegetables or making sheet-pan meals.
3. Saucepan & Stockpot: For cooking grains, soups, and broths.
4. Non-Toxic Skillet (Stainless steel or ceramic-coated): For sautéing proteins and vegetables.
5. Blender or Food Processor: For smoothies, sauces, and dips.
6. Storage Containers: Glass or BPA-free plastic for storing prepped ingredients and meals.
7. Slow Cooker or Instant Pot (Optional but helpful): Set it and forget it—great for busy days.

Pro Tip: Label your containers with meal names and prep dates using masking tape and a marker. It keeps your fridge and freezer organized and reduces waste.

Reading Labels and Shopping Smart

Understanding food labels is a crucial skill—especially when managing Graves' disease. Many packaged foods contain hidden ingredients that can worsen inflammation or trigger symptoms.

Watch Out For:

- Hidden sugars: Look for names like high-fructose corn syrup, cane juice, dextrose, maltodextrin.
- Processed oils: Avoid hydrogenated oils, corn oil, soybean oil.
- Artificial additives: MSG, food dyes, artificial sweeteners like aspartame or sucralose.
- Gluten (if sensitive): Watch for wheat, barley, rye, malt, brewer's yeast.

Smart Shopping Tips:

- Shop the perimeter of the store—this is where fresh produce, meats, and whole foods are found.
- Choose items with 5 ingredients or fewer.
- Look for certifications like "gluten-free," "non-GMO," or "organic" when applicable.
- Buy in bulk when possible (especially grains, nuts, and seeds) to save money and reduce packaging waste.

Reminder: Just because something is labeled "natural" or "healthy" doesn't mean it's thyroid-friendly. Always read the fine print.

Managing Food Sensitivities

Food sensitivities can worsen symptoms like brain fog, fatigue, digestive issues, and skin problems. While sensitivities are individual, those with Graves' disease are more likely to develop sensitivities due to increased gut permeability (aka "leaky gut")—a common autoimmune companion.

Common Triggers:

- Gluten
- Dairy
- Soy
- Eggs
- Corn
- Nightshades (tomatoes, peppers, eggplant, potatoes—for some)

How to Identify Sensitivities:

1. Elimination Diet: Temporarily remove common trigger foods for 3–4 weeks, then reintroduce them one at a time, tracking symptoms.
2. Food Journal: Note what you eat and how you feel for 1–2 weeks. Look for patterns (e.g., bloating, headaches, mood changes).
3. Work with a Functional Medicine Practitioner: If you're unsure where to start, a professional can help guide testing and analysis.
1. How to Manage Them:
2. Find alternatives you enjoy: Almond milk instead of cow's milk, gluten-free pasta, coconut yogurt, etc.
3. Prepare meals at home so you know exactly what's in your food.
4. Use simple, whole-food recipes to minimize additives and allergens.

Note: Managing sensitivities isn't about restriction—it's about discovery. Once you know what works for your body, eating becomes empowering.

Creating a thyroid-friendly kitchen isn't about perfection—it's about preparation. With a thoughtfully stocked pantry, smart tools, and time-saving habits, you're building a lifestyle that supports healing from the inside out.

You don't need to do it all at once. Start small. Pick one strategy this week: maybe batch-cook grains, prep some veggies, or invest in a good knife. Every intentional step you take makes the next one easier.

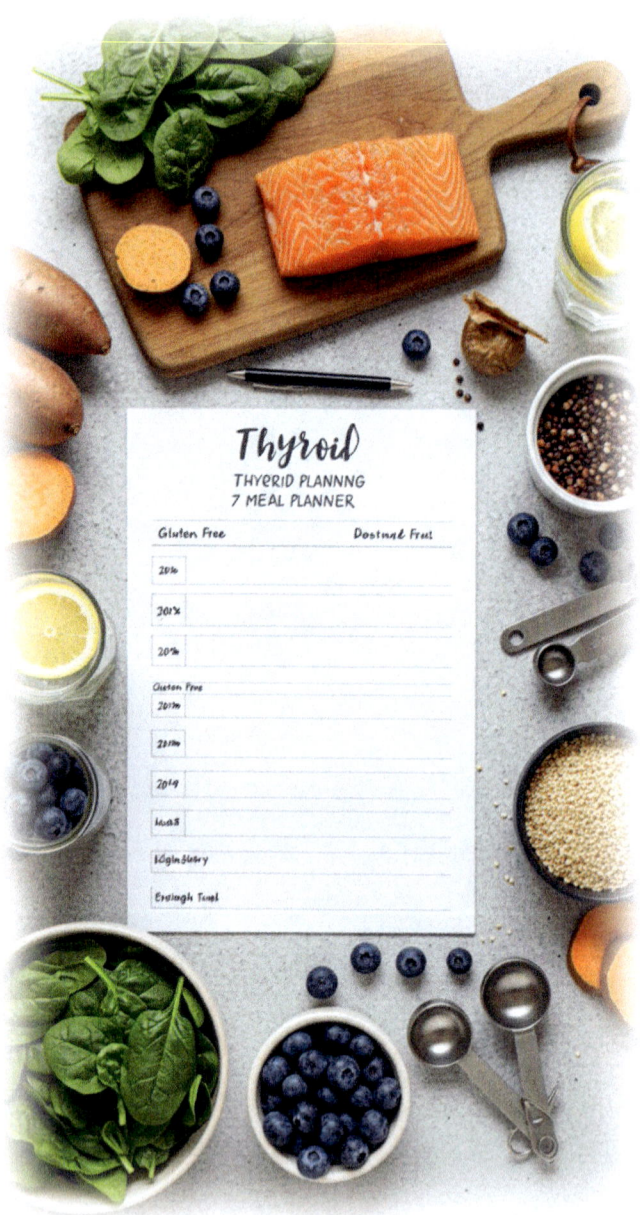

CHAPTER 4:

YOUR 28-DAY MEAL PLAN FOR THYROID HEALING

Healing through food isn't about deprivation—it's about nourishment, balance, and consistency. This 28-day meal plan is designed to reduce inflammation, stabilize energy, and support your thyroid function with nutrient-dense meals you'll actually enjoy. Think of it as your personal roadmap to feeling better, one meal at a time.

Let's start with Week 1, where we focus on building a solid foundation.

Week 1: Shopping List

To make grocery shopping simple, here's everything you'll need for Week 1 based on the recipes in this book.

Produce:

- Leafy greens (spinach, kale, arugula)

- Broccoli
- Carrots
- Sweet potatoes
- Bell peppers (red, yellow, or green)
- Avocados
- Cucumbers
- Zucchini
- Berries (blueberries, raspberries, strawberries)
- Bananas
- Apples
- Garlic
- Onions
- Fresh herbs (cilantro, parsley, basil)
- Lemons

Proteins & Dairy Alternatives:

- Free-range eggs
- Organic chicken breast
- Wild-caught salmon
- Grass-fed beef
- Canned tuna (in olive oil or water)
- Unsweetened coconut yogurt
- Almond or coconut milk

Healthy Fats & Oils:

- Extra virgin olive oil
- Avocado oil

- Coconut oil
- Raw almonds and walnuts
- Pumpkin seeds
- Chia seeds
- Ground flaxseeds

Pantry Staples:

- Quinoa
- Brown rice
- Gluten-free oats
- Chickpeas
- Lentils
- Canned coconut milk
- Dark chocolate (70% or higher)
- Apple cider vinegar
- Tahini
- Honey or maple syrup
- Cinnamon, turmeric, ginger, black pepper

Week 1: Meal Prep Guidelines

A little prep goes a long way! Here's how to set yourself up for success:

1. Batch Cook Proteins: Grill or bake chicken breasts and salmon fillets for easy meal assembly.
2. Prepare Grains in Advance: Cook a large batch of quinoa and brown rice for quick meals.
3. Make a Smoothie Prep Bag: Freeze berries, spinach, and bananas in portions for easy morning smoothies.
4. Chop Vegetables: Store chopped carrots, cucumbers, and bell peppers in airtight containers for quick salads and snacks.
5. Roast Vegetables: Roast sweet potatoes and broccoli for easy side dishes.
6. Soak Nuts and Seeds: Pre-soaking nuts and seeds improves digestibility and nutrient absorption.

Week 1: Meal Plan

Day 1

- Breakfast: Pumpkin Seed Trail Mix + Coconut Yogurt Parfait
- Lunch: Grilled Chicken with Roasted Sweet Potatoes & Broccoli

- Snack: Cucumber & Hummus Bites
- Dinner: One-Pan Salmon with Quinoa & Steamed Greens

Day 2

- Breakfast: Avocado Cocoa Mousse + Herbal Tea
- Lunch: Quinoa Salad with Chickpeas, Cucumber & Lemon Dressing
- Snack: Carrot Cake Bliss Balls
- Dinner: Baked Pears with Walnuts & Cinnamon + Wild-Caught Salmon

Day 3

- Breakfast: Thyroid-Supporting Smoothie Bowl
- Lunch: Lentil & Vegetable Soup
- Snack: Fig & Nut Bars
- Dinner: Garlic Herb Chicken with Zucchini Noodles

Day 4

- Breakfast: Spiced Quinoa Pudding
- Lunch: Tuna Salad with Avocado & Greens
- Snack: Golden Milk Bites
- Dinner: Sweet Potato & Tahini Cookies + Grilled Salmon

Day 5

- Breakfast: Almond Butter Oatmeal with Berries
- Lunch: Quinoa-Stuffed Bell Peppers
- Snack: Coconut Yogurt Parfait
- Dinner: Roasted Chicken with Lemon & Herbs

Day 6

- Breakfast: Carrot Cake Bliss Balls + Green Smoothie
- Lunch: Brown Rice & Chickpea Bowl with Tahini Dressing
- Snack: Pumpkin Seed Trail Mix
- Dinner: Garlic Shrimp with Steamed Vegetables

Day 7

- Breakfast: Sweet Potato Hash with Eggs
- Lunch: Grilled Chicken & Spinach Salad with Olive Oil Dressing
- Snack: Cucumber & Hummus Bites
- Dinner: One-Pan Baked Fish with Lemon & Herbs

Adapting The Plan to Your Needs

Life happens, and flexibility is key. If you need to switch a meal, swap with another from the same category (e.g., swap one smoothie for another). Not a fan of a specific ingredient? Substitute with a thyroid-friendly alternative, like swapping quinoa for brown rice or salmon for chicken.

Tracking Your Progress

Keep a simple food and symptom journal to monitor how your body responds to the meal plan. Write down:

1. How you feel after each meal
2. Any digestive issues, energy dips, or improvements
3. Changes in sleep, mood, and overall well-being
4. After a week, review your notes to identify patterns and make adjustments.

Adjusting For Symptom Flares

If you experience symptom flares (like fatigue, heart palpitations, or digestive distress), consider:

1. Reducing inflammatory foods (limit dairy, sugar, and processed snacks).
2. Drinking more herbal teas like ginger or chamomile.
3. Prioritizing easy-to-digest meals (soups, broths, and smoothies).
4. Adding more omega-3s from fish or flaxseeds to calm inflammation.

Week 2: Building Consistency and Balance

You've completed your first week—amazing! By now, you might be noticing small but powerful shifts, like steadier energy levels, better digestion, or even improved mood. In Week 2, we continue reinforcing these positive changes with another set of delicious, nutrient-dense meals designed to help your thyroid thrive.

Week 2: Shopping List

Produce:

- Leafy greens (spinach, kale, romaine)
- Cauliflower
- Sweet potatoes
- Carrots

- Zucchini
- Bell peppers
- Avocados
- Cucumbers
- Tomatoes
- Berries (blueberries, raspberries, blackberries)
- Bananas
- Apples
- Garlic
- Onions
- Fresh herbs (basil, parsley, cilantro)
- Lemons

Proteins & Dairy Alternatives:

- Free-range eggs
- Organic chicken thighs
- Wild-caught cod or tilapia
- Grass-fed beef
- Canned wild salmon
- Unsweetened almond or coconut milk
- Unsweetened coconut yogurt

Healthy Fats & Oils:

- Extra virgin olive oil
- Avocado oil
- Raw walnuts
- Cashews

- Pumpkin seeds
- Chia seeds
- Ground flaxseeds

Pantry Staples:

- Quinoa
- Brown rice
- Gluten-free oats
- Lentils
- Chickpeas
- Canned coconut milk
- Dark chocolate (70% or higher)
- Apple cider vinegar
- Tahini
- Honey or maple syrup
- Cinnamon, turmeric, ginger, black pepper

Week 2: Meal Prep Guidelines

A little meal prep can help you stay on track and avoid last-minute unhealthy choices. Here's what you can prepare in advance:

1. Batch Cook Proteins: Grill or bake chicken and cod for easy use throughout the week.
2. Cook a Large Batch of Quinoa: Store in the fridge for quick meals.

3. Chop and Store Veggies: Have pre-cut zucchini, bell peppers, and cucumbers ready for salads and sides.
4. Make a Breakfast Base: Pre-make Spiced Quinoa Pudding or Thyroid-Supporting Smoothie Bags for quick morning meals.
5. Prepare a Nut & Seed Mix: Combine walnuts, pumpkin seeds, and flaxseeds for a nutrient-rich snack topping.

Week 2: Meal Plan

Day 8

- Breakfast: Almond Butter Oatmeal with Berries
- Lunch: Roasted Cauliflower & Chickpea Bowl
- Snack: No-Bake Fig & Nut Bars
- Dinner: Grilled Chicken with Lemon & Quinoa

Day 9

- Breakfast: Green Smoothie with Chia Seeds
- Lunch: Spinach & Lentil Soup
- Snack: Cucumber & Hummus Bites
- Dinner: Garlic Herb Cod with Roasted Sweet Potatoes

Day 10
- Breakfast: Coconut Yogurt Parfait with Berries
- Lunch: Quinoa Salad with Avocado & Pumpkin Seeds
- Snack: Carrot Cake Bliss Balls
- Dinner: Lemon-Tahini Chicken with Steamed Greens

Day 11
- Breakfast: Spiced Quinoa Pudding
- Lunch: Brown Rice & Grilled Salmon Bowl
- Snack: Pumpkin Seed Trail Mix
- Dinner: Garlic Shrimp with Zucchini Noodles

Day 12
- Breakfast: Sweet Potato Hash with Eggs
- Lunch: Quinoa-Stuffed Bell Peppers
- Snack: Golden Milk Bites
- Dinner: Balsamic Chicken with Roasted Vegetables

Day 13
- Breakfast: Thyroid-Supporting Smoothie Bowl
- Lunch: Spinach & Avocado Salad with Lemon Dressing

- Snack: Dark Chocolate & Walnut Bites
- Dinner: Lentil & Carrot Stew

Day 14

- Breakfast: Chia Pudding with Fresh Berries
- Lunch: Chickpea & Tomato Soup
- Snack: No-Bake Fig & Nut Bars
- Dinner: One-Pan Baked Fish with Garlic & Herbs

Adapting The Plan to Your Needs

Feeling too full? Reduce portion sizes and listen to your body's cues. Need more variety? Swap in another recipe from the book that fits your cravings while keeping it thyroid-friendly.

Tracking Your Progress

Continue keeping a food and symptom journal. Pay attention to:

1. Energy levels throughout the day
2. Sleep quality and mood changes
3. Any digestive symptoms or improvements
4. Noting these patterns helps fine-tune your diet for what works best for your body.

Adjusting For Symptom Flares

If you experience any symptom flares this week, consider:

1. Reducing raw cruciferous vegetables like cauliflower and kale (lightly steaming them can help).
2. Drinking more ginger or peppermint tea to ease digestion.
3. Ensuring you're eating balanced meals with enough protein and healthy fats.

WEEK 3: DEEPENING THE HEALING PROCESS

By now, you might be noticing positive shifts—perhaps fewer energy crashes, improved digestion, or better focus. Week 3 is all about maintaining momentum while introducing new flavors and nutrient-dense meals that continue to support your thyroid function.

Week 3: Shopping List

Produce:

- Leafy greens (spinach, arugula, kale)
- Brussels sprouts
- Carrots
- Beets
- Zucchini
- Bell peppers
- Avocados
- Cucumbers
- Tomatoes
- Sweet potatoes
- Berries (blueberries, strawberries, raspberries)
- Apples
- Bananas
- Garlic
- Onions
- Fresh herbs (cilantro, basil, parsley)
- Lemons

Proteins & Dairy Alternatives:

- Free-range eggs
- Organic chicken breast
- Wild-caught cod or salmon
- Grass-fed beef
- Canned tuna (in olive oil or water)
- Unsweetened almond or coconut milk
- Unsweetened coconut yogurt

Healthy Fats & Oils:

- Extra virgin olive oil
- Avocado oil
- Raw almonds
- Chia seeds
- Pumpkin seeds
- Walnuts

Pantry Staples:

- Quinoa
- Brown rice
- Gluten-free oats
- Lentils
- Chickpeas
- Canned coconut milk
- Dark chocolate (70% or higher)
- Apple cider vinegar
- Tahini
- Honey or maple syrup
- Cinnamon, turmeric, ginger, black pepper

Week 3: Meal Prep Guidelines

This week, try focusing on variety while still keeping meal prep simple. Here are some ways to streamline your cooking:

1. Batch Cook Proteins: Prepare grilled chicken and baked fish to use throughout the week.
2. Make a Soup or Stew: Cook a batch of Lentil & Carrot Stew for quick lunches or dinners.
3. Chop & Store Veggies: Have sliced cucumbers, bell peppers, and beets ready for salads and sides.
4. Cook a Grain Base: Prepare quinoa or brown rice for easy meal assembly.
5. Prepare a Nut & Seed Mix: Combine walnuts, pumpkin seeds, and flaxseeds for a nutrient-rich snack topping.

Week 3: Meal Plan

Day 15

- Breakfast: Spiced Quinoa Pudding
- Lunch: Roasted Brussels Sprouts & Quinoa Bowl
- Snack: Cucumber & Hummus Bites
- Dinner: Lemon Herb Chicken with Roasted Beets

Day 16

- Breakfast: Coconut Yogurt Parfait with Berries
- Lunch: Lentil & Vegetable Soup

- Snack: Dark Chocolate & Walnut Bites
- Dinner: Garlic Shrimp with Zucchini Noodles

Day 17

- Breakfast: Thyroid-Supporting Smoothie Bowl
- Lunch: Avocado & Chickpea Salad with Lemon Dressing
- Snack: Golden Milk Bites
- Dinner: Roasted Salmon with Sweet Potato Mash

Day 18

- Breakfast: Almond Butter Oatmeal with Berries
- Lunch: Quinoa-Stuffed Bell Peppers
- Snack: Pumpkin Seed Trail Mix
- Dinner: Garlic Herb Cod with Steamed Greens

Day 19

- Breakfast: Chia Pudding with Fresh Berries
- Lunch: Brown Rice & Grilled Chicken Bowl
- Snack: Carrot Cake Bliss Balls
- Dinner: Balsamic Chicken with Roasted Vegetables

Day 20

- Breakfast: Green Smoothie with Chia Seeds
- Lunch: Spinach & Avocado Salad with Lemon Dressing
- Snack: No-Bake Fig & Nut Bars
- Dinner: Lentil & Carrot Stew

Day 21

- Breakfast: Sweet Potato Hash with Eggs
- Lunch: Chickpea & Tomato Soup
- Snack: Coconut Yogurt Parfait
- Dinner: One-Pan Baked Fish with Lemon & Herbs

Adapting The Plan to Your Needs

Feel free to adjust portion sizes based on your hunger levels. If a recipe doesn't appeal to you, swap it with another from the book while keeping it thyroid-friendly.

Tracking Your Progress

As you enter Week 3, keep an eye on:

1. Whether your energy levels are more stable throughout the day
2. Any improvements in digestion and gut health
3. How your sleep quality and mood are shifting

4. Your food and symptom journal will continue to be a useful tool for identifying patterns.

Adjusting For Symptom Flares

If you notice a flare-up of symptoms, you might try:

1. Focusing on lighter meals (soups, stews, and smoothies)
2. Reducing inflammatory foods like excessive raw vegetables or high-sugar snacks
3. Drinking herbal teas like chamomile or ginger to support digestion

Week 4: Sustaining Your Progress for Long-Term Health

You've made it to the final week of the plan! By now, you've built habits that support your thyroid health, discovered new favorite meals, and learned how food impacts your symptoms. This last week focuses on keeping your momentum going while reinforcing the foundations of your healing journey.

Week 4: Shopping List

Produce:

- Leafy greens (spinach, kale, romaine)
- Broccoli
- Carrots
- Zucchini
- Bell peppers
- Avocados
- Cucumbers
- Tomatoes
- Sweet potatoes
- Berries (blueberries, blackberries, strawberries)
- Apples
- Bananas
- Garlic
- Onions
- Fresh herbs (parsley, cilantro, basil)
- Lemons

Proteins & Dairy Alternatives:

- Free-range eggs
- Organic chicken thighs
- Wild-caught salmon or cod
- Grass-fed beef
- Canned wild tuna
- Unsweetened almond or coconut milk
- Unsweetened coconut yogurt

Healthy Fats & Oils:

- Extra virgin olive oil
- Avocado oil
- Raw walnuts
- Chia seeds
- Pumpkin seeds
- Cashews

Pantry Staples:

- Quinoa
- Brown rice
- Lentils
- Chickpeas
- Canned coconut milk
- Dark chocolate (70% or higher)
- Apple cider vinegar
- Tahini
- Honey or maple syrup
- Cinnamon, turmeric, ginger, black pepper

Week 4: Meal Prep Guidelines

You're likely more comfortable with meal prepping by now, so this week's focus is efficiency. Here's how to stay ahead:

1. Batch Cook Proteins: Roast chicken and bake salmon for easy meals.

2. Prepare a Big Salad Base: Chop greens, cucumbers, and bell peppers for quick lunches.
3. Cook a Grain in Advance: Have quinoa or brown rice ready for simple meal assembly.
4. Make a Soup: A batch of Chickpea & Tomato Soup can serve as a quick, warm meal.
5. Pre-Blend Smoothie Bags: Portion out ingredients for thyroid-supporting smoothies.

Week 4: Meal Plan

Day 22

- Breakfast: Green Smoothie with Chia Seeds
- Lunch: Roasted Veggie & Quinoa Bowl
- Snack: Almond Butter & Apple Slices
- Dinner: Garlic Herb Chicken with Steamed Greens

Day 23

- Breakfast: Chia Pudding with Fresh Berries
- Lunch: Spinach & Avocado Salad with Lemon Dressing
- Snack: Pumpkin Seed Trail Mix

- Dinner: Baked Salmon with Sweet Potato Mash

Day 24

- Breakfast: Spiced Quinoa Pudding
- Lunch: Chickpea & Tomato Soup
- Snack: No-Bake Fig & Nut Bars
- Dinner: Grilled Shrimp with Zucchini Noodles

Day 25

- Breakfast: Thyroid-Supporting Smoothie Bowl
- Lunch: Quinoa-Stuffed Bell Peppers
- Snack: Dark Chocolate & Walnut Bites
- Dinner: Lemon-Tahini Chicken with Roasted Carrots

Day 26

- Breakfast: Sweet Potato Hash with Eggs
- Lunch: Lentil & Avocado Salad
- Snack: Golden Milk Bites
- Dinner: One-Pan Garlic Cod with Steamed Broccoli

Day 27

- Breakfast: Coconut Yogurt Parfait with Berries

- Lunch: Brown Rice & Grilled Chicken Bowl
- Snack: Carrot Cake Bliss Balls
- Dinner: Roasted Salmon with Quinoa & Spinach

Day 28

- Breakfast: Almond Butter Oatmeal with Berries
- Lunch: Spinach & Chickpea Salad with Lemon Dressing
- Snack: Dark Chocolate & Walnut Bites
- Dinner: Lentil & Carrot Stew

Adapting The Plan to Your Needs

Now that you're at the end of the 28 days, reflect on what meals worked best for you. Keep your favorite recipes in rotation and adjust as needed based on your personal preferences and symptom response.

Tracking Your Progress

At this stage, take time to:

1. Review your food and symptom journal. What meals made you feel your best?
2. Notice if your energy levels, digestion, and mood have improved.

3. Celebrate your wins—big or small!

Adjusting For Symptom Flares

If symptoms arise, don't stress. Continue focusing on whole, nutrient-dense foods, stay hydrated, and listen to your body. Herbal teas, gentle movement, and stress management can all help bring balance.

Moving Forward

Completing this meal plan isn't the end of your journey—it's the beginning of a long-term, sustainable approach to eating for thyroid health. You now have the tools and knowledge to continue making nourishing choices that support your well-being. Keep experimenting with recipes, listening to your body, and enjoying the process!

In the next chapter, we'll get to the heart of the matter—recipes! You'll find delicious, nourishing meals designed to support your thyroid, calm your immune system, and make you feel good in your body again.

Ready to cook your way to healing? Let's go!

BREAKFAST RECIPES

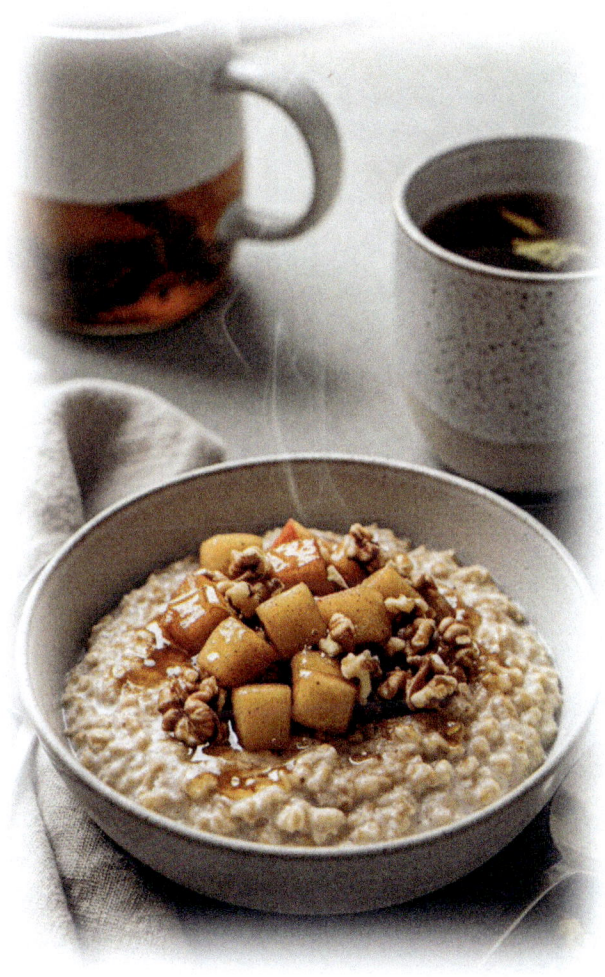

Sweet Potato & Avocado Hash

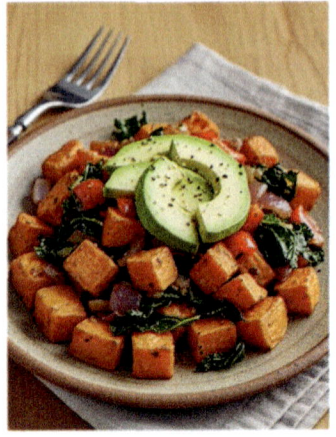

Prep Time: 10 minutes

Cook Time: 20 minutes

Serving Size: 2 servings

Nutritional Value (per serving):

Calories: 320 | Protein: 7g | Carbs: 35g | Fat: 18g | Fiber: 8g

Ingredients:

- 1 large sweet potato, peeled and diced
- 1 tablespoon olive oil
- ½ red onion, chopped
- 1 bell pepper, diced
- 1 teaspoon cumin
- ½ teaspoon turmeric
- Salt and pepper to taste
- 1 ripe avocado, sliced
- Fresh parsley for garnish

Instructions:

1. Heat olive oil in a skillet over medium heat. Add diced sweet potato and cook for 10 minutes, stirring occasionally.
2. Add onion, bell pepper, cumin, turmeric, salt, and pepper. Cook until vegetables are soft and

lightly browned, about 10 more minutes.
3. Remove from heat. Plate and top with sliced avocado and fresh parsley.

> **Expert Tip:**
>
> *For added protein, top with a poached egg or sprinkle with pumpkin seeds—rich in zinc for thyroid support.*

Sweet potatoes are a fantastic source of slow-digesting carbohydrates and vitamin A, which supports immune health and reduces inflammation—key factors in managing Graves' disease.

Chia & Flaxseed Overnight Pudding

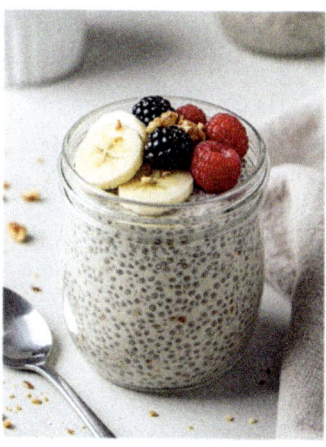

Prep Time: 5 minutes

Chill Time: At least 4 hours (overnight recommended)

Serving Size: 2 servings

Nutritional Value (per serving):

Calories: 280 | Protein: 8g | Carbs: 20g | Fat: 18g | Fiber: 10g

Ingredients:

- 2 tablespoons chia seeds
- 1 tablespoon ground flaxseed
- 1 cup unsweetened almond milk
- ½ teaspoon vanilla extract
- 1 teaspoon maple syrup (optional)
- Fresh berries and chopped almonds for topping

Instructions:

1. In a jar or bowl, mix chia seeds, flaxseed, almond milk, vanilla, and maple syrup.
2. Stir well and refrigerate for at least 4 hours or overnight.
3. In the morning, stir again and top with berries and almonds.

Expert Tip:

Add a sprinkle of cinnamon to help stabilize blood sugar and reduce thyroid flare-ups.

Chia and flaxseeds are rich in omega-3 fatty acids, which help reduce inflammation and regulate hormonal balance.

Zinc-Powered Pumpkin Seed Smoothie Bowl

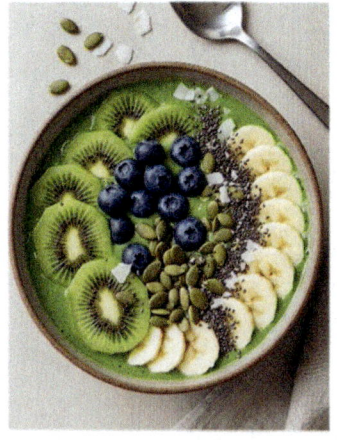

Prep Time: 10 minutes

Cook Time: None

Serving Size: 1 large bowl or 2 small

Nutritional Value (per serving):

Calories: 360 | Protein: 12g | Carbs: 28g | Fat: 22g | Fiber: 6g

Ingredients:

- 1 frozen banana
- ½ cup frozen blueberries
- ½ avocado
- 1 tablespoon pumpkin seeds
- 1 tablespoon almond butter
- 1 cup unsweetened coconut milk
- 1 teaspoon chia seeds (for topping)
- Coconut flakes or granola (optional topping)

Instructions:

1. Blend all ingredients (except toppings) until smooth and creamy.
2. Pour into a bowl and top with chia seeds,

coconut flakes, or granola.

Expert Tip:

Add a scoop of clean, plant-based protein powder to boost your protein intake—essential for hormone production.

Pumpkin seeds are one of the best sources of zinc, a crucial mineral for immune regulation and thyroid hormone conversion.

Savory Quinoa Breakfast Bowl

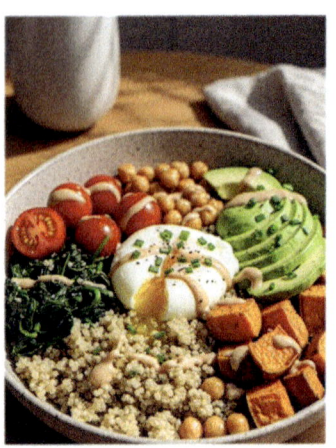

Prep Time: 10 minutes

Cook Time: 15 minutes

Serving Size: 2 bowls

Nutritional Value (per serving):

Calories: 390 | Protein: 14g | Carbs: 35g | Fat: 20g | Fiber: 6g

Ingredients:

- 1 cup cooked quinoa
- 1 tablespoon olive oil
- 1 cup baby spinach
- ½ cup cherry tomatoes, halved
- ¼ cup shredded carrots
- 1 boiled egg (optional)
- Sea salt and pepper to taste
- Avocado slices for topping

Expert Tip:

Make a large batch of quinoa at the beginning of the week for easy breakfast bowls and lunch salads.

Instructions:

1. Warm olive oil in a skillet, sauté spinach, tomatoes, and carrots until soft (about 5 minutes).
2. Stir in cooked quinoa and season with salt and pepper.
3. Divide into bowls and top with avocado slices and boiled egg, if using.

Quinoa is a complete protein, packed with essential amino acids and magnesium, supporting nervous system function and sustained energy.

Thyroid-Loving Berry Almond Smoothie

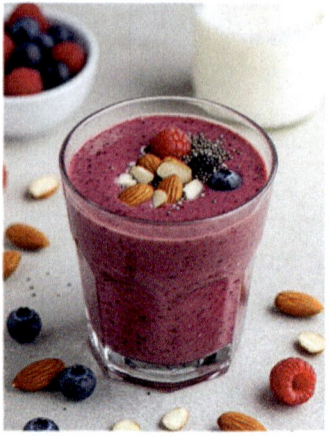

Prep Time: 5 minutes

Cook Time: None

Serving Size: 1 smoothie

Nutritional Value (per serving):

Calories: 290 | Protein: 10g | Carbs: 26g | Fat: 17g | Fiber: 7g

Ingredients:

- 1 cup mixed frozen berries
- 1 tablespoon almond butter
- 1 tablespoon ground flaxseed
- ½ cup unsweetened almond milk
- ½ cup plain coconut yogurt
- ½ teaspoon cinnamon

Instructions:

1. Blend all ingredients until smooth.
2. Pour into a glass and enjoy immediately.

Expert Tip:

Add a few Brazil nuts to the blend for an extra selenium boost (but keep it to 1–2 to avoid excessive intake).

This smoothie combines antioxidant-rich berries with selenium-packed almonds, supporting immune health and reducing oxidative stress in the thyroid.

Coconut Millet Porridge with Berries

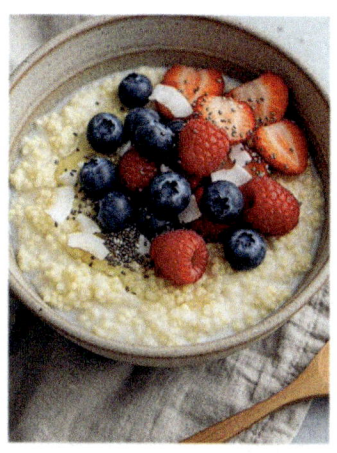

Prep Time: 5 minutes

Cook Time: 20 minutes

Serving Size: 2 servings

Nutritional Value (per serving):

Calories: 330 | Protein: 7g | Carbs: 38g | Fat: 16g | Fiber: 5g

Ingredients:

- ½ cup uncooked millet
- 1 cup water
- ½ cup full-fat coconut milk
- 1 teaspoon cinnamon
- 1 teaspoon maple syrup (optional)
- ½ cup mixed berries (fresh or thawed)
- 1 tablespoon chopped walnuts or almonds

Instructions:

1. In a saucepan, bring millet and water to a boil. Reduce to a simmer and cook for 15–20 minutes until soft.
2. Stir in coconut milk, cinnamon, and maple syrup (if using). Simmer for 2 more minutes.
3. Serve warm topped with berries and chopped nuts.

Expert Tip:

Soak the millet overnight to speed up cooking time and improve nutrient absorption.

Millet is a naturally gluten-free grain that's gentle on the digestive system. When paired with healthy fats from coconut milk and antioxidant-rich berries, it becomes a nourishing and grounding breakfast for thyroid balance.

Almond Flour Pancakes with Wild Blueberry Compote

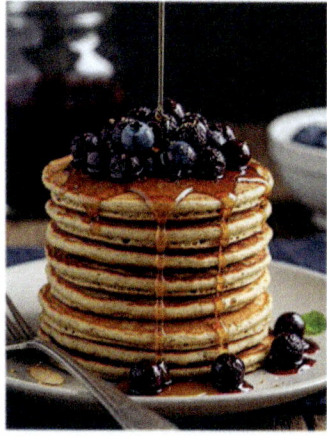

Prep Time: 10 minutes

Cook Time: 10 minutes

Serving Size: 2 servings (makes about 4 pancakes)

Nutritional Value (per serving):

Calories: 310 | Protein: 10g | Carbs: 22g | Fat: 21g | Fiber: 4g

Ingredients:

- 1 cup almond flour
- 2 eggs
- ¼ cup unsweetened almond milk
- ½ teaspoon baking soda
- ½ teaspoon vanilla extract
- Pinch of sea salt
- Wild Blueberry Compote:
- ½ cup wild blueberries (frozen or fresh)
- 1 teaspoon lemon juice
- ½ teaspoon maple syrup (optional)

Instructions:

1. Whisk together pancake ingredients in a bowl until smooth.
2. Heat a non-stick skillet over medium heat. Pour batter to form small pancakes, cooking 2–3 minutes per side.
3. In a small saucepan, heat blueberries, lemon juice, and maple syrup until bubbling. Mash slightly and simmer for 3–4 minutes.
4. Top pancakes with warm compote.

These gluten-free pancakes use almond flour, rich in selenium and healthy fats, and are naturally low in carbohydrates. The blueberry compote adds a punch of antioxidants to support immune health.

Expert Tip:

Wild blueberries contain higher levels of antioxidants than regular blueberries—great for reducing thyroid-related oxidative stress.

Veggie-Packed Breakfast Muffins (Gluten-Free)

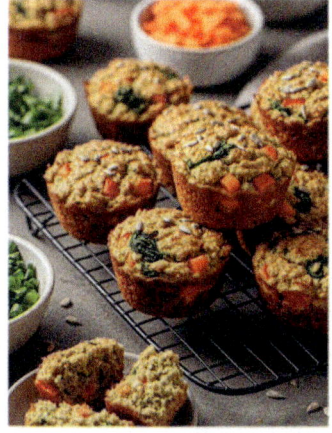

Prep Time: 15 minutes

Cook Time: 25 minutes

Serving Size: 6 muffins (3 servings)

Nutritional Value (per 2 muffins):

Calories: 270 | Protein: 11g | Carbs: 12g | Fat: 19g | Fiber: 3g

Ingredients:

- 4 eggs
- ½ cup unsweetened almond milk
- ½ cup finely chopped spinach
- ¼ cup grated zucchini
- ¼ cup chopped red bell pepper
- ¼ cup almond flour
- 1 tablespoon ground flaxseed
- ½ teaspoon turmeric
- Salt and pepper to taste

Instructions:

1. Preheat oven to 350°F (175°C) and grease a muffin tin or use silicone liners.
2. In a bowl, whisk together eggs and almond milk.

3. Add all veggies, almond flour, flaxseed, turmeric, salt, and pepper. Mix well.
4. Pour mixture evenly into muffin cups and bake for 20–25 minutes or until set.
5. Cool slightly before serving or store in the fridge.

Expert Tip:

Add a sprinkle of nutritional yeast before baking for a cheesy flavor and an extra B-vitamin boost.

These savory muffins are perfect for meal prep and packed with fiber, protein, and antioxidants to help stabilize energy and mood throughout the day.

Creamy Avocado & Greens Smoothie

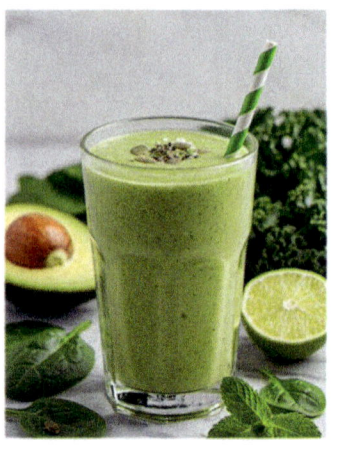

Prep Time: 5 minutes

Cook Time: None

Serving Size: 1 smoothie

Nutritional Value (per serving):

Calories: 310 | Protein: 8g | Carbs: 18g | Fat: 22g | Fiber: 8g

Ingredients:

- ½ ripe avocado
- 1 cup spinach or kale
- 1 small green apple, chopped
- ½ cucumber
- Juice of ½ lemon
- 1 cup unsweetened coconut water or almond milk
- 1 tablespoon chia seeds

Instructions:

1. Blend all ingredients until smooth.
2. Adjust liquid as needed for desired consistency. Serve chilled.

Expert Tip:

Blend with a few ice cubes and mint leaves for a refreshing, hydrating twist—great for hot days or post-exercise recovery.

Avocados provide healthy monounsaturated fats, fiber, and potassium. Combined with leafy greens, this smoothie supports detoxification and thyroid hormone transport.

Buckwheat Banana Breakfast Bowl

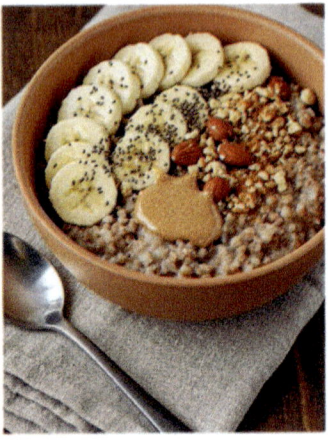

Prep Time: 10 minutes

Cook Time: 15 minutes

Serving Size: 2 bowls

Nutritional Value (per serving):

Calories: 340 | Protein: 9g | Carbs: 40g | Fat: 14g | Fiber: 6g

Ingredients:

- ½ cup raw buckwheat groats
- 1 cup water
- ½ cup unsweetened almond milk
- 1 ripe banana, mashed
- 1 teaspoon cinnamon
- 1 tablespoon flaxseed meal
- 1 tablespoon almond butter
- Sliced banana and chopped walnuts for topping

Instructions:

1. Rinse buckwheat thoroughly and cook in water until tender (10–15 minutes).
2. Stir in almond milk, mashed banana, cinnamon, and flaxseed. Simmer for 2 minutes.

3. Serve warm with almond butter, sliced banana, and chopped walnuts on top.

calm the nervous system and supports hormone regulation.

Expert Tip:

Soaking buckwheat overnight before cooking makes it easier to digest and reduces cooking time.

Despite its name, buckwheat is gluten-free and rich in magnesium—a key mineral that helps

MAIN DISHES

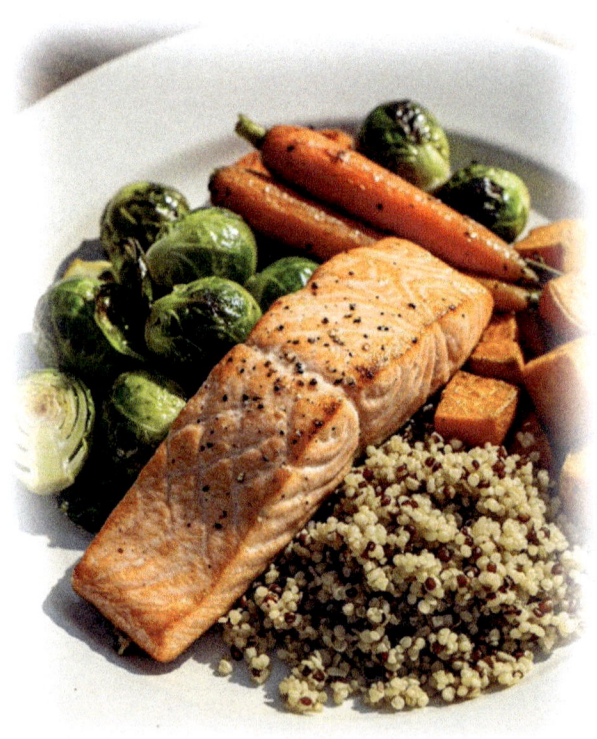

Lemon Herb Baked Salmon with Quinoa and Steamed Greens

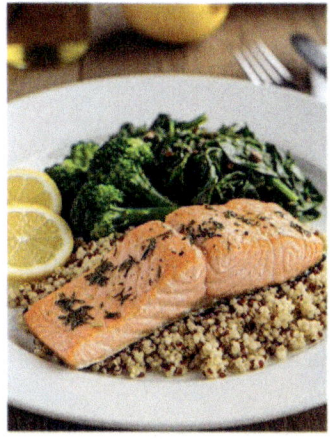

Prep Time: 10 minutes

Cook Time: 20 minutes

Serving Size: 2 servings

Nutritional Value (per serving):

Calories: 410 | Protein: 32g | Carbs: 25g | Fat: 22g | Fiber: 5g

Ingredients:

- 2 salmon fillets (4–6 oz each)
- Juice of 1 lemon
- 1 tablespoon olive oil
- 1 teaspoon dried oregano
- Salt and pepper to taste
- 1 cup cooked quinoa
- 2 cups steamed spinach or kale

Instructions:

1. Preheat oven to 375°F (190°C).
2. Place salmon fillets on a lined baking dish. Drizzle with lemon juice and olive oil, then sprinkle with

oregano, salt, and pepper.
3. Bake for 15–20 minutes until the fish flakes easily.
4. Serve over a bed of quinoa with a side of steamed greens.

Expert Tip:

For added zinc, garnish with toasted pumpkin seeds right before serving.

Salmon is an excellent source of omega-3 fatty acids and selenium—two key nutrients that support thyroid hormone production and reduce inflammation.

Turmeric Chicken and Veggie Stir-Fry

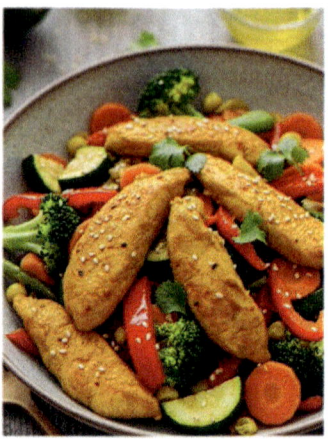

Prep Time: 15 minutes

Cook Time: 15 minutes

Serving Size: 2–3 servings

Nutritional Value (per serving):

Calories: 390 | Protein: 30g | Carbs: 20g | Fat: 22g | Fiber: 4g

Ingredients:

1. 2 boneless skinless chicken breasts, sliced
2. 1 tablespoon coconut oil or avocado oil
3. 1 red bell pepper, sliced
4. 1 zucchini, sliced
5. 1 cup broccoli florets
6. 1 clove garlic, minced
7. 1 teaspoon turmeric
8. ½ teaspoon ginger
9. Salt to taste
10. 1 tablespoon coconut aminos or low-sodium tamari

Instructions:

1. Heat oil in a large skillet over medium heat. Add chicken and cook until browned.
2. Add garlic, turmeric, and ginger. Stir to coat.
3. Add vegetables and stir-fry for 5–7 minutes until tender-crisp.
4. Add coconut aminos, stir well, and cook for another 2 minutes.

Expert Tip:

Serve over cauliflower rice for a low-carb option that supports blood sugar balance.

This anti-inflammatory stir-fry is rich in color,

nutrients, and thyroid-friendly spices. Turmeric helps reduce autoimmune activity and supports liver detox.

Lentil and Sweet Potato Shepherd's Pie (Vegan)

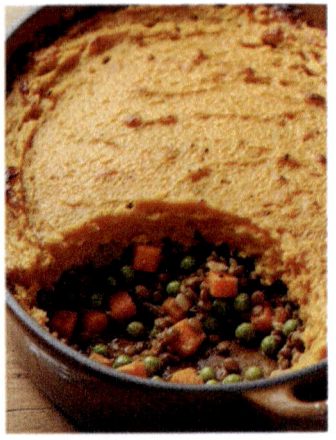

Prep Time: 20 minutes

Cook Time: 25 minutes

Serving Size: 4 servings

Nutritional Value (per serving):

Calories: 420 | Protein: 16g | Carbs: 50g | Fat: 14g | Fiber: 10g

Ingredients:

Filling:

- 1 tablespoon olive oil
- 1 small onion, chopped
- 1 carrot, diced
- 1 celery stalk, diced
- 2 cloves garlic, minced
- 1 cup cooked green or brown lentils
- 1 tablespoon tomato paste
- ½ cup vegetable broth
- 1 teaspoon dried thyme
- Salt and pepper to taste

Topping:

- 2 medium sweet potatoes, peeled and chopped
- 1 tablespoon olive oil or coconut oil
- 1 tablespoon unsweetened almond milk

Instructions:

1. Boil sweet potatoes until soft, about 15 minutes. Drain and mash with oil and almond milk. Set aside.
2. Meanwhile, heat olive oil in a skillet. Sauté onion, carrot, and celery for 5–7 minutes. Add garlic and cook 1 more minute.
3. Stir in lentils, tomato paste, broth, thyme, salt, and pepper. Simmer for 5 minutes until thickened.
4. Spoon lentil filling into a baking dish and top with mashed sweet potatoes.
5. Bake at 375°F (190°C) for 20 minutes until golden.

Ginger Garlic Cod with Bok Choy and Brown Rice

Expert Tip:

Sprinkle with hemp seeds before serving for an extra protein and omega-3 boost.

Packed with fiber, iron, and plant-based protein, this comforting dish supports digestive health and stabilizes energy—important for those managing thyroid fatigue

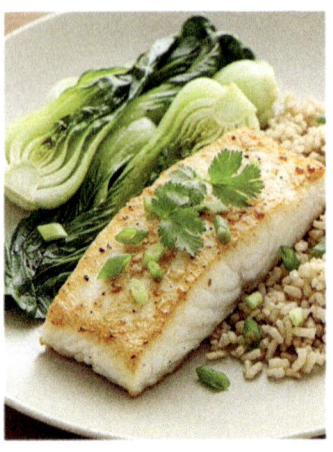

Prep Time: 10 minutes

Cook Time: 15 minutes

Serving Size: 2 servings

Nutritional Value (per serving):

Calories: 360 | Protein: 28g | Carbs: 30g | Fat: 14g | Fiber: 4g

Ingredients:

- 2 cod fillets
- 1 tablespoon sesame oil
- 2 teaspoons grated fresh ginger
- 2 cloves garlic, minced
- 1 tablespoon coconut aminos
- 1 tablespoon lime juice
- 2 cups bok choy, chopped
- 1 cup cooked brown rice

Instructions:

1. Heat sesame oil in a skillet. Add garlic and ginger, sauté for 1 minute.
2. Add cod fillets and cook for 3–4 minutes per side, or until cooked through.
3. Remove cod and add bok choy to the skillet. Stir-fry for 2–3 minutes.
4. Return cod to pan, add coconut aminos and lime juice. Heat for 1 more minute.
5. Serve with brown rice.

Expert Tip:

Drizzle with a touch of tahini before serving for healthy fats and added flavor.

Cod is a lean source of protein and selenium, while bok choy adds fiber and calcium to support bone health and digestion—two common areas of concern in Graves' disease.

Chickpea and Spinach Coconut Curry

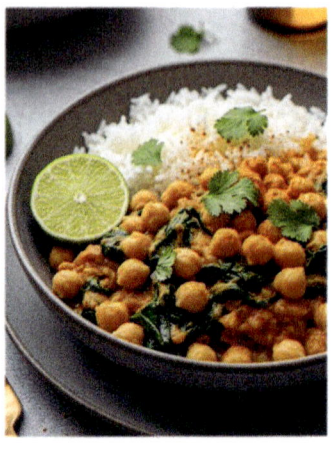

Prep Time: 10 minutes

Cook Time: 20 minutes

Serving Size: 3–4 servings

Nutritional Value (per serving):

Calories: 390 | Protein: 14g | Carbs: 35g | Fat: 22g | Fiber: 8g

Ingredients:

- 1 tablespoon coconut oil
- 1 small onion, diced
- 2 cloves garlic, minced
- 1 tablespoon curry powder
- 1 teaspoon ground cumin
- 1 can (15 oz) chickpeas, drained and rinsed
- 1 can (14 oz) full-fat coconut milk
- 2 cups baby spinach
- Salt and pepper to taste
- Fresh cilantro for garnish

Instructions:

1. Heat coconut oil in a large skillet over medium heat. Add onion and sauté until soft.
2. Add garlic, curry powder, and cumin. Stir for 1 minute.
3. Add chickpeas and coconut milk. Simmer for 10 minutes.
4. Stir in spinach and cook until wilted.
5. Garnish with cilantro and serve with quinoa or gluten-free flatbread.

Expert Tip:

For a calcium boost, stir in a handful of chopped cooked kale with the spinach.

This plant-based curry is rich in fiber, protein, and anti-inflammatory spices that support gut health and hormone metabolism—two crucial pillars for managing Graves' symptoms.

Baked Chicken Thighs with Roasted Root Vegetables

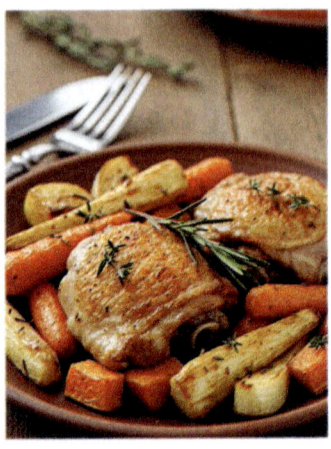

Prep Time: 15 minutes

Cook Time: 35 minutes

Serving Size: 4 servings

Nutritional Value (per serving):

Calories: 460 | Protein: 28g | Carbs: 24g | Fat: 28g | Fiber: 5g

Ingredients:

- 4 bone-in, skin-on chicken thighs
- 2 tablespoons olive oil
- 1 teaspoon dried rosemary
- 1 teaspoon garlic powder
- Salt and pepper to taste
- 1 cup chopped carrots
- 1 cup chopped sweet potatoes
- 1 cup chopped parsnips or beets

Instructions:

1. Preheat oven to 400°F (200°C).
2. In a large bowl, toss chicken thighs with olive oil, rosemary, garlic powder, salt, and pepper.
3. Spread root vegetables on a sheet pan. Drizzle with olive oil and season with salt and pepper.
4. Place chicken thighs on top of vegetables.
5. Roast for 35–40 minutes, or until chicken is golden and cooked through.

Expert Tip:

Save the chicken bones to make a homemade bone broth rich in collagen and minerals—great for gut and thyroid support.

Dark meat chicken provides more zinc and iron than white meat—both essential for immune and thyroid health. Pairing it with antioxidant-rich root vegetables creates a satisfying and balanced meal

Zucchini Noodle Bowl with Sesame Turkey Meatballs

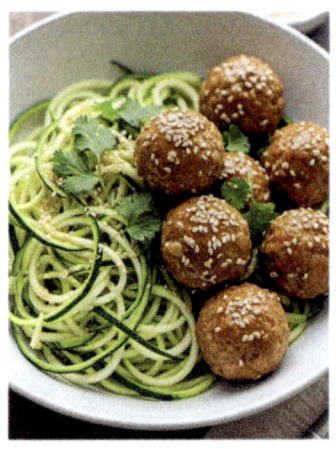

Prep Time: 20 minutes

Cook Time: 20 minutes

Serving Size: 3–4 servings

Nutritional Value (per serving):

Calories: 350 | Protein: 26g | Carbs: 12g | Fat: 22g | Fiber: 3g

Ingredients:

Meatballs:

- 1 lb ground turkey
- 1 tablespoon sesame oil
- 1 teaspoon garlic powder
- 1 teaspoon ground ginger
- 1 tablespoon coconut aminos
- 1 tablespoon finely chopped scallions
- Pinch of salt
- Zoodle Bowl:
- 3 medium zucchinis, spiralized
- 1 tablespoon sesame oil
- 1 teaspoon rice vinegar
- 1 teaspoon coconut aminos
- Sesame seeds and chopped cilantro for garnish

Instructions:

1. Preheat oven to 375°F (190°C). Mix meatball ingredients in a bowl. Form into 1-inch balls and place on a lined baking tray.
2. Bake for 18–20 minutes until fully cooked.
3. In a large skillet, heat sesame oil. Add spiralized zucchini and sauté for 3–4 minutes.
4. Stir in rice vinegar and coconut aminos.
5. Serve meatballs over zucchini noodles, garnished with sesame seeds and cilantro.

Black Bean and Quinoa Stuffed Peppers

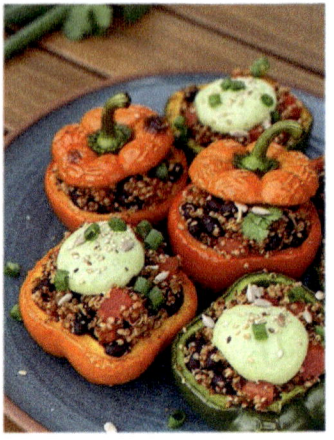

Expert Tip:

Add a pinch of kelp flakes to boost iodine naturally— only if you've been cleared by your healthcare provider to include it.

This low-carb, high-protein meal is light but nourishing. Turkey is a lean source of selenium and zinc, and zucchini noodles are easy on the digestive system and packed with fiber.

Prep Time: 15 minutes

Cook Time: 30 minutes

Serving Size: 4 servings

Nutritional Value (per serving):

Calories: 410 | Protein: 17g | Carbs: 45g | Fat: 18g | Fiber: 10g

Ingredients:

1. 4 large bell peppers, halved and deseeded
2. 1 tablespoon olive oil
3. 1 small onion, diced
4. 2 cloves garlic, minced
5. 1 teaspoon cumin
6. 1 teaspoon smoked paprika
7. 1 cup cooked quinoa
8. 1 cup black beans, rinsed and drained
9. ½ cup diced tomatoes (no salt added)
10. Salt and pepper to taste

Instructions:

1. Preheat oven to 375°F (190°C).
2. Sauté onion and garlic in olive oil over medium heat until soft. Add spices, quinoa, black beans, and tomatoes. Stir and heat through.
3. Fill pepper halves with the mixture and place in a baking dish.
4. Add ¼ cup water to the dish and cover with foil. Bake for 25–30 minutes.
5. Garnish with chopped parsley or avocado slices.

Expert Tip:

Use tri-colored quinoa for added antioxidants and visual appeal.

This plant-based meal is a complete protein source

thanks to the quinoa and black beans combo. It's rich in fiber and magnesium, which help regulate metabolism and support adrenal function.

One-Pan Mediterranean Chicken and Vegetables

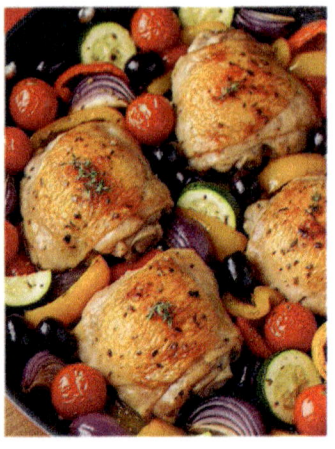

Prep Time: 15 minutes

Cook Time: 30 minutes

Serving Size: 4 servings

Nutritional Value (per serving):

Calories: 430 | Protein: 32g | Carbs: 18g | Fat: 26g | Fiber: 5g

Ingredients:

- 4 boneless chicken thighs or breasts
- 2 tablespoons olive oil
- 1 zucchini, sliced
- 1 red bell pepper, sliced
- 1 red onion, chopped
- 1 cup cherry tomatoes
- ¼ cup Kalamata olives, halved
- 1 teaspoon oregano
- Salt and pepper to taste

Instructions:

1. Preheat oven to 400°F (200°C).
2. In a large mixing bowl, combine all ingredients and toss to coat.
3. Spread everything onto a sheet pan in a single layer.
4. Roast for 25–30 minutes, stirring once halfway through.

Expert Tip:

Add a handful of arugula or spinach after baking for a boost of thyroid-friendly greens.

This dish is loaded with thyroid-supporting nutrients like vitamin C, selenium, and healthy fats. The olives and olive oil provide monounsaturated fats to reduce inflammation.

Butternut Squash and Kale Risotto (Dairy-Free)

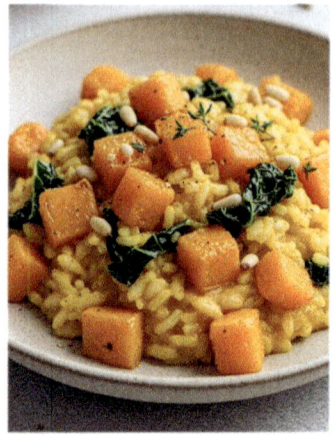

Prep Time: 15 minutes

Cook Time: 30 minutes

Serving Size: 4 servings

Nutritional Value (per serving):

Calories: 380 | Protein: 10g | Carbs: 50g | Fat: 15g | Fiber: 6g

Ingredients:

- 1 tablespoon olive oil
- 1 small onion, chopped
- 1 clove garlic, minced
- 1 cup arborio rice
- 2½ cups low-sodium vegetable broth (warmed)
- 1 cup cubed butternut squash
- 1 cup chopped kale
- 1 tablespoon nutritional yeast (optional)
- Salt and pepper to taste

Instructions:

1. In a saucepan, heat olive oil over medium heat. Sauté onion and garlic until soft.
2. Add rice and stir to coat, then add squash.

3. Gradually add warm broth ½ cup at a time, stirring constantly until absorbed.
4. Continue for about 25 minutes until rice is tender and creamy.
5. Stir in kale and nutritional yeast. Cook another 2–3 minutes. Season to taste.

Expert Tip:

Stir in a splash of almond milk for extra creaminess without the dairy.

A comforting yet nourishing meal, this risotto skips dairy but doesn't skimp on flavor. Butternut squash provides vitamin A and antioxidants, while kale adds iron and fiber.

Grilled Miso-Ginger Salmon with Cucumber Salad

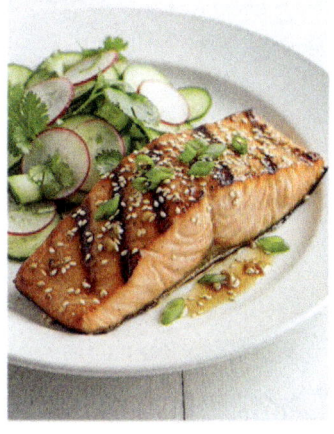

Prep Time: 15 minutes (plus 30 minutes to marinate)

Cook Time: 10 minutes

Serving Size: 2 servings

Nutritional Value (per serving):

Calories: 400 | Protein: 35g | Carbs: 10g | Fat: 25g | Fiber: 2g

Ingredients:

Miso-Ginger Salmon:

- 2 salmon fillets (4–6 oz each)
- 1 tablespoon white miso paste (use reduced sodium)
- 1 tablespoon rice vinegar
- 1 tablespoon grated ginger
- 1 teaspoon sesame oil

Cucumber Salad:

- 1 cucumber, thinly sliced
- 1 teaspoon rice vinegar
- 1 teaspoon sesame oil
- Pinch of sea salt
- Toasted sesame seeds (for garnish)

Instructions:

1. Mix miso, vinegar, ginger, and sesame oil in a bowl. Coat salmon and marinate for 30 minutes in the fridge.
2. Grill or pan-sear salmon over medium-high heat for 4–5 minutes per side, until fully cooked.
3. Toss cucumber with vinegar, sesame oil, and salt. Let sit for 10 minutes.
4. Serve salmon with cucumber salad and a sprinkle of sesame seeds.

Expert Tip:

Always check with your doctor before consuming fermented soy like miso. If sensitive, swap with coconut aminos and extra ginger for a similar flavor.

Salmon is rich in omega-3s and selenium, while miso (in moderation) provides beneficial probiotics. This light and refreshing dish is perfect for supporting immune and thyroid health without overloading the digestive system.

Baked Falafel with Tahini Sauce and Cabbage Slaw

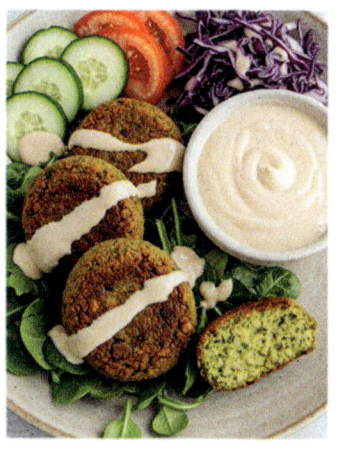

Prep Time: 20 minutes

Cook Time: 25 minutes

Serving Size: 4 servings (2–3 falafel per serving)

Nutritional Value (per serving):

Calories: 370 | Protein: 14g | Carbs: 30g | Fat: 20g | Fiber: 8g

Ingredients:

Falafel:

- 1½ cups cooked chickpeas
- ¼ cup chopped parsley
- 1 clove garlic
- 1 tablespoon lemon juice
- 1 teaspoon cumin
- 1 teaspoon coriander
- 2 tablespoons oat flour (gluten-free)
- Salt to taste
- 2 tablespoons olive oil (for brushing)

Slaw:

- 1 cup shredded red cabbage
- 1 teaspoon olive oil
- 1 teaspoon apple cider vinegar

Sauce:

- 2 tablespoons tahini
- 1 tablespoon lemon juice
- 2 tablespoons water
- Pinch of salt

Instructions:

1. Preheat oven to 375°F (190°C).
2. Blend falafel ingredients in a food processor until crumbly but moist. Form into small patties.
3. Place on a lined baking sheet, brush with olive oil, and bake for 25 minutes, flipping halfway.
4. Mix slaw ingredients and whisk tahini sauce until smooth.

5. Serve falafel over slaw with a drizzle of tahini sauce.

Expert Tip:

Add a handful of spinach to the falafel mix to increase iron and magnesium content.

These baked falafels are full of fiber, plant-based protein, and anti-inflammatory herbs. Served with a simple cabbage slaw, this meal is gut-friendly and naturally gluten-free.

Cauliflower Rice Stir-Fry with Shrimp and Vegetables

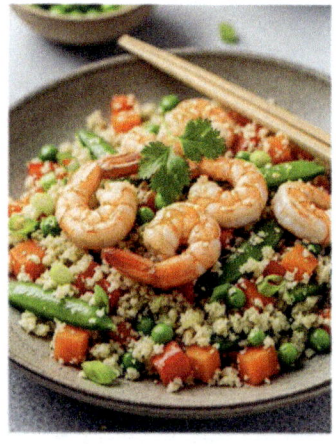

Prep Time: 15 minutes

Cook Time: 15 minutes

Serving Size: 2–3 servings

Nutritional Value (per serving):

Calories: 310 | Protein: 26g | Carbs: 14g | Fat: 18g | Fiber: 4g

Ingredients:

- 1 tablespoon avocado oil
- ½ lb shrimp, peeled and deveined
- 2 cups cauliflower rice
- 1 carrot, julienned
- ½ red bell pepper, sliced
- 2 scallions, chopped
- 1 clove garlic, minced
- 1 tablespoon coconut aminos
- ½ teaspoon grated fresh ginger
- Salt and pepper to taste

Instructions:

1. Heat oil in a large skillet. Add shrimp, garlic, and ginger. Cook until shrimp is pink, about 3–4 minutes.
2. Remove shrimp and sauté veggies until tender, about 5 minutes.
3. Add cauliflower rice and coconut aminos. Stir well and cook another 3 minutes.
4. Return shrimp to pan, heat through, and season to taste.

Expert Tip:

For added selenium, toss in a few chopped Brazil nuts just before serving (use sparingly—1–2 nuts per serving).

Shrimp is a great source of iodine and protein, while

cauliflower rice keeps this dish light and blood sugar-friendly. A perfect quick weeknight dinner that supports thyroid metabolism.

Stuffed Acorn Squash with Wild Rice and Cranberries

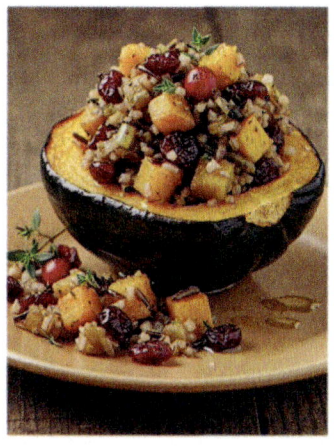

Prep Time: 20 minutes

Cook Time: 40 minutes

Serving Size: 2 servings

Nutritional Value (per serving):

Calories: 420 | Protein: 10g | Carbs: 60g | Fat: 16g | Fiber: 9g

Ingredients:

- 1 medium acorn squash, halved and seeded
- 1 tablespoon olive oil
- Salt and pepper to taste
- 1 cup cooked wild rice
- ¼ cup dried unsweetened cranberries
- 2 tablespoons chopped walnuts
- 1 tablespoon chopped parsley
- 1 teaspoon maple syrup (optional)

Instructions:

1. Preheat oven to 400°F (200°C). Brush squash halves with olive oil, season with salt and pepper, and bake cut-side down for 30–35 minutes until tender.
2. In a bowl, combine rice, cranberries, walnuts, parsley, and maple syrup.
3. Flip squash halves over and fill with the rice mixture. Return to oven for 5–10 minutes.
4. Serve warm, garnished with extra herbs if desired.

Expert Tip:

You can swap acorn squash with delicata squash for a slightly quicker cook time and thinner skin.

A seasonal, antioxidant-rich dish that supports thyroid and immune health. Wild rice provides zinc and fiber, while acorn squash delivers vitamin C and carotenoids.

Coconut Chickpea Shakshuka (Egg-Free Option)

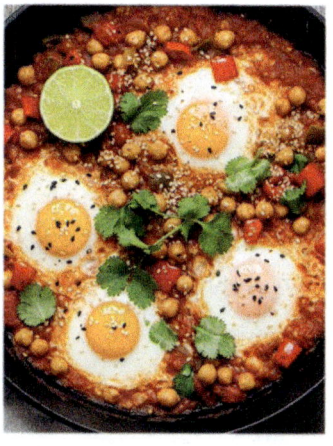

Prep Time: 10 minutes

Cook Time: 20 minutes

Serving Size: 3–4 servings

Nutritional Value (per serving):

Calories: 360 | Protein: 12g | Carbs: 30g | Fat: 22g | Fiber: 7g

Ingredients:

- 1 tablespoon olive oil
- 1 onion, chopped
- 1 bell pepper, chopped
- 2 cloves garlic, minced
- 1 teaspoon cumin
- 1 teaspoon smoked paprika
- 1 can (14 oz) diced tomatoes
- ½ can full-fat coconut milk
- 1 can (15 oz) chickpeas, drained
- Salt and pepper to taste
- Fresh parsley for garnish

Instructions:

1. Heat olive oil in a skillet. Sauté onion, garlic, and bell pepper until soft.
2. Stir in cumin, paprika, and tomatoes. Simmer for 5 minutes.
3. Add coconut milk and chickpeas. Simmer uncovered for 10–15 minutes until thickened.
4. Season and garnish with parsley.

Expert Tip:

For a non-vegan version, crack 2–3 eggs over the mixture and cover with a lid for 6–8 minutes until the whites are set.

Inspired by the traditional dish but made thyroid-friendly and vegan, this version uses coconut milk for richness and chickpeas for protein. It's warming, anti-inflammatory, and packed with flavor.

From My Heart to Yours

If this book has brought you comfort, clarity, or even just one recipe you love—I'd be truly grateful if you'd take a moment to leave a review on Amazon.

Simply scan the QR code to share your thoughts

Your words not only support my work but also help others on their healing journey.

With gratitude,

Thalia Rowen

And if you ever have questions, need guidance, or just want to share your experience, feel free to reach out to me directly at thaliarowenbooks@gmail.com. I'd love to hear from you and be part of your healing journey.

Thank you so much for your support!

SIDES, SALADS, AND SOUPS

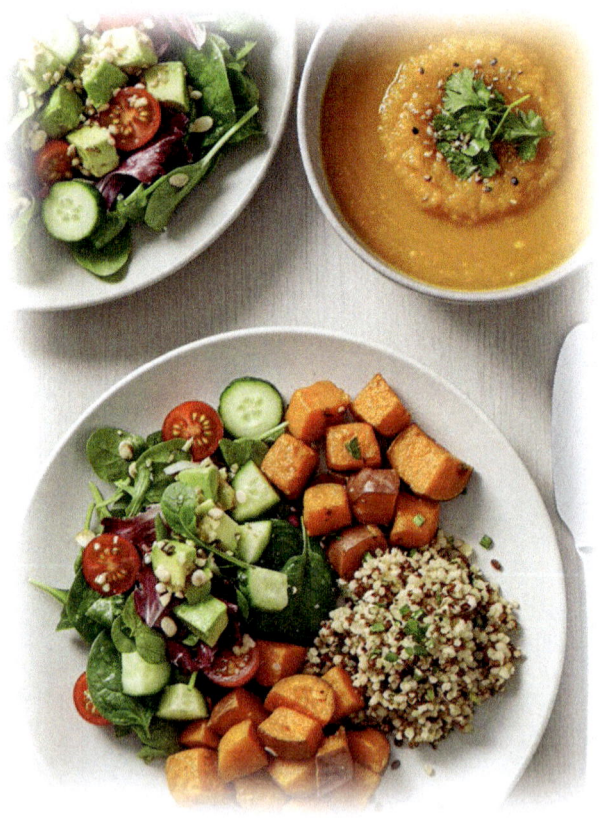

Roasted Rainbow Vegetables with Thyme

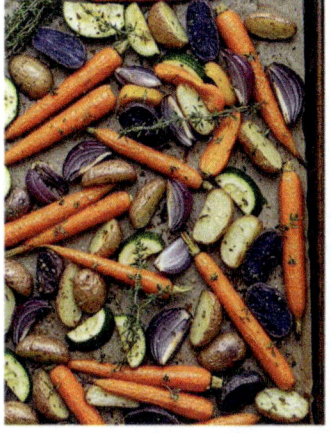

Prep Time: 10 minutes

Cook Time: 30 minutes

Serving Size: 4 servings

Nutritional Value (per serving):

Calories: 150 | Carbs: 18g | Protein: 3g | Fat: 8g | Fiber: 6g

Ingredients:

- 1 cup chopped carrots
- 1 cup chopped sweet potatoes
- 1 cup chopped zucchini
- 1 red bell pepper, chopped
- 1 tablespoon olive oil
- 1 teaspoon fresh thyme (or ½ tsp dried)
- Salt and pepper to taste

Instructions:

1. Preheat oven to 400°F (200°C).
2. In a large bowl, toss all vegetables with olive oil, thyme, salt, and pepper.
3. Spread evenly on a baking sheet and roast for 25–30 minutes, stirring halfway through.

4. Serve warm as a colorful side.

Expert Tip:

Use a mix of colors—orange, green, red, and purple—to maximize phytonutrients that help reduce inflammation and support thyroid function.

Colorful vegetables are packed with antioxidants, vitamins, and minerals that support immune and thyroid health. Roasting brings out their natural sweetness and flavor, making this a perfect side for any meal.

Quinoa and Kale Power Bowl

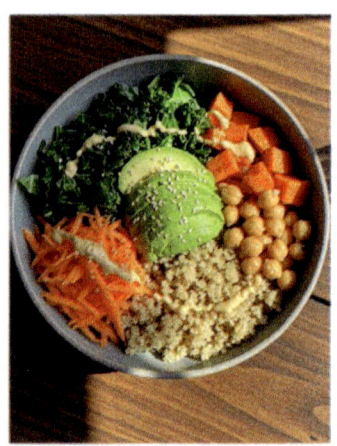

Prep Time: 15 minutes

Cook Time: 15 minutes

Serving Size: 2–3 servings

Nutritional Value (per serving):

Calories: 280 | Carbs: 35g | Protein: 9g | Fat: 11g | Fiber: 6g

Ingredients:

- 1 cup cooked quinoa
- 1 cup chopped kale, massaged
- ½ cup shredded carrot
- ¼ cup chopped cucumber
- 2 tablespoons olive oil
- 1 tablespoon lemon juice
- 1 teaspoon Dijon mustard
- Salt and pepper to taste

Instructions:

1. Cook quinoa according to package instructions and let cool slightly.
2. In a bowl, combine olive oil, lemon juice, mustard, salt, and pepper to make a dressing.
3. Toss quinoa with kale, carrots, and cucumber. Drizzle with dressing and mix well.
4. Serve warm or chilled.

Expert Tip:

Massage kale with a bit of olive oil before adding—it softens the leaves and enhances digestion.

This grain dish is packed with plant-based protein, fiber, magnesium, and antioxidants—all beneficial for hormonal and metabolic balance in Graves' Disease.

Creamy Carrot Ginger Soup

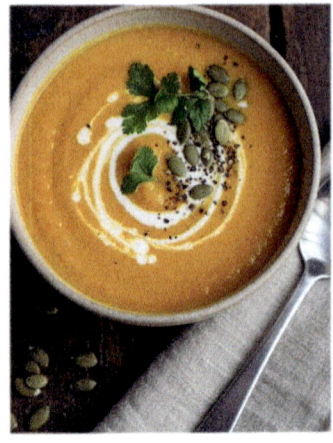

Prep Time: 10 minutes

Cook Time: 25 minutes

Serving Size: 4 servings

Nutritional Value (per serving):

Calories: 180 | Carbs: 20g | Protein: 3g | Fat: 10g | Fiber: 4g

Ingredients:

1. 1 tablespoon olive oil
2. 1 onion, chopped
3. 4 cups chopped carrots
4. 1 tablespoon grated fresh ginger
5. 3 cups low-sodium vegetable broth
6. ½ cup full-fat coconut milk
7. Salt and pepper to taste

Instructions:

1. Heat olive oil in a pot and sauté onions until soft.
2. Add carrots and ginger, cook for 5 minutes.
3. Pour in broth, bring to a boil, then reduce to simmer for 20 minutes.

4. Blend soup until smooth. Stir in coconut milk and season to taste.
5. Serve warm with a drizzle of extra coconut milk if desired.

Expert Tip:

For added zinc and selenium, sprinkle ground pumpkin seeds or hemp seeds on top before serving.

Ginger is a natural anti-inflammatory and digestive aid, while carrots are rich in beta-carotene. This soup is soothing and perfect for thyroid-friendly comfort food.

Beet and Arugula Salad with Lemon Vinaigrette

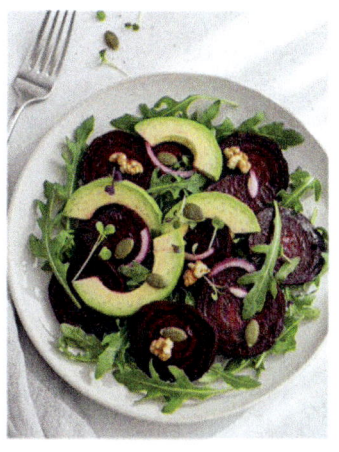

Prep Time: 15 minutes

Cook Time: 0 minutes (use pre-cooked beets if desired)

Serving Size: 2–3 servings

Nutritional Value (per serving):

Calories: 220 | Carbs: 16g | Protein: 4g | Fat: 15g | Fiber: 5g

Ingredients:

- 2 cups arugula
- 1 cup cooked and sliced beets
- 2 tablespoons walnuts
- 1 tablespoon hemp seeds
- 2 teaspoons olive oil
- 1 tablespoon lemon juice
- ½ teaspoon Dijon mustard
- Salt and pepper to taste

Instructions:

1. Arrange arugula on plates, top with sliced beets, walnuts, and hemp seeds.
2. In a small jar, shake together olive oil, lemon juice, mustard, salt, and pepper.
3. Drizzle over salad and serve immediately.

Expert Tip:

Add a few slices of avocado for extra healthy fats and creaminess without dairy.

Beets are liver-supportive and help with detox, while arugula provides a peppery kick and supports digestion. This salad is bright, flavorful, and thyroid-friendly.

Healing Turmeric Lentil Soup

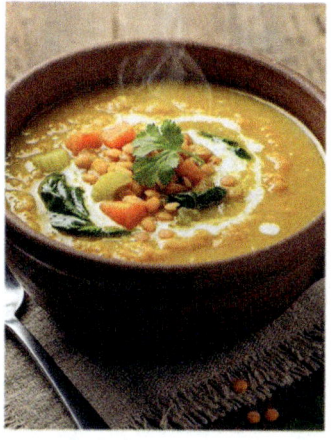

Prep Time: 10 minutes

Cook Time: 30 minutes

Serving Size: 4 servings

Nutritional Value (per serving):

Calories: 300 | Carbs: 36g | Protein: 14g | Fat: 10g | Fiber: 10g

Ingredients:

- 1 tablespoon coconut oil or olive oil
- 1 onion, chopped
- 2 cloves garlic, minced
- 1 teaspoon ground turmeric
- 1 teaspoon cumin
- 1 cup red lentils, rinsed
- 4 cups vegetable broth
- 1 carrot, chopped
- 1 celery stalk, chopped
- Salt and pepper to taste
- Fresh cilantro or parsley (optional)

Instructions:

1. Heat oil in a large pot. Sauté onion and garlic until translucent.
2. Stir in turmeric and cumin. Add lentils, carrot, celery, and broth.

3. Bring to a boil, then reduce heat and simmer for 25–30 minutes, until lentils are soft.
4. Season with salt and pepper. Garnish with fresh herbs.

Expert Tip:

Add a squeeze of lemon just before serving to enhance flavor and aid in iron absorption.

Lentils are rich in plant-based protein and iron, while turmeric offers strong anti-inflammatory benefits. This soup is grounding, healing, and perfect for a thyroid-supportive reset.

Sweet Potato and Chickpea Salad with Tahini Dressing

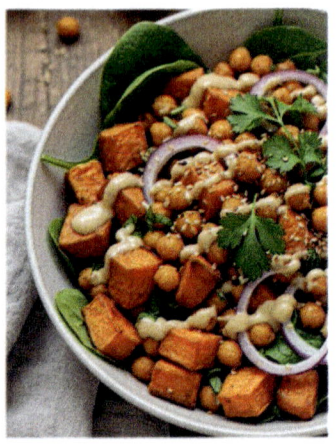

Prep Time: 10 minutes

Cook Time: 25 minutes

Serving Size: 4 servings

Nutritional Value (per serving):

Calories: 320 | Carbs: 40g | Protein: 10g | Fat: 14g | Fiber: 9g

Ingredients:

- 2 medium sweet potatoes, peeled and cubed
- 1 cup cooked chickpeas (or canned, drained and rinsed)
- 2 tablespoons olive oil
- 4 cups mixed greens or spinach
- 2 tablespoons tahini
- 1 tablespoon lemon juice
- 1 tablespoon water (as needed to thin dressing)
- ½ teaspoon garlic powder
- Salt and pepper to taste

Instructions:

1. Preheat oven to 400°F (200°C). Toss sweet potatoes with olive oil, salt, and pepper, then roast for 20–25 minutes until tender.
2. In a small bowl, whisk tahini, lemon juice, garlic powder, and water until smooth.
3. In a large bowl, combine roasted sweet potatoes, chickpeas, and greens. Drizzle with tahini dressing and toss to coat.
4. Serve warm or chilled.

Expert Tip:

For a boost of selenium, sprinkle with sunflower or pumpkin seeds just before serving.

Sweet potatoes are rich in complex carbs and vitamin A, while chickpeas provide plant-based protein and fiber. This hearty salad is a perfect lunch or side to support stable energy and thyroid function.

Garlic Sautéed Green Beans and Mushrooms

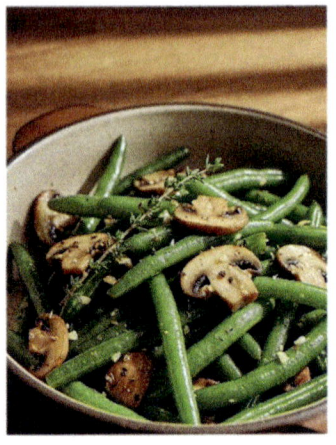

Prep Time: 5 minutes

Cook Time: 12 minutes

Serving Size: 4 servings

Nutritional Value (per serving):

Calories: 110 | Carbs: 10g | Protein: 3g | Fat: 7g | Fiber: 4g

Ingredients:

- 2 cups green beans, trimmed
- 1 cup sliced mushrooms (cremini or button)
- 1 tablespoon olive oil
- 2 cloves garlic, minced
- Salt and black pepper to taste
- 1 teaspoon lemon zest (optional)

Instructions:

1. Heat olive oil in a skillet over medium heat.
2. Add garlic and cook for 30 seconds, then add green beans and mushrooms.
3. Sauté for about 10–12 minutes, stirring often, until vegetables are tender.
4. Season with salt, pepper, and lemon zest before serving.

Expert Tip:

Don't overcook green beans—keeping them crisp helps retain nutrients and adds great texture.

This simple yet flavorful side features green beans rich in vitamins C and K, and mushrooms that support immune function. A great low-effort, nutrient-dense dish.

Mediterranean Millet Salad

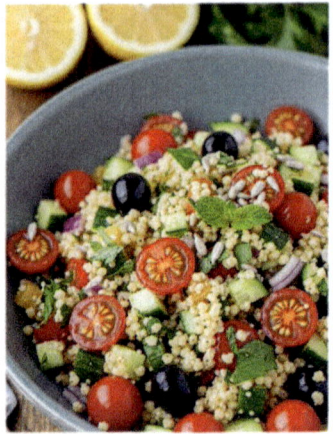

Prep Time: 15 minutes

Cook Time: 20 minutes

Serving Size: 4 servings

Nutritional Value (per serving):

Calories: 260 | Carbs: 34g | Protein: 7g | Fat: 10g | Fiber: 5g

Ingredients:

- 1 cup cooked millet
- 1 cup cherry tomatoes, halved
- ½ cucumber, diced
- ¼ cup chopped parsley
- 2 tablespoons kalamata olives, sliced
- 2 tablespoons olive oil
- Juice of ½ lemon
- Salt and pepper to taste

Instructions:

1. Cook millet according to package instructions. Let it cool.
2. In a bowl, combine all ingredients and toss well.
3. Serve at room temperature or chilled.

Expert Tip:

Make a large batch and store in the fridge—it keeps well for 3–4 days and makes a quick lunch!

Millet is a gluten-free ancient grain that supports digestion and provides key nutrients like magnesium and phosphorus. Combined with Mediterranean flavors, it makes a refreshing and energizing dish.

Broccoli and Cauliflower Soup

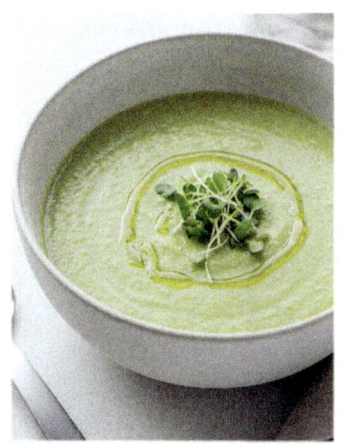

Prep Time: 10 minutes

Cook Time: 25 minutes

Serving Size: 4 servings

Nutritional Value (per serving):

Calories: 190 | Carbs: 18g | Protein: 5g | Fat: 11g | Fiber: 5g

Ingredients:

- 1 tablespoon olive oil
- 1 onion, chopped
- 2 cups broccoli florets
- 2 cups cauliflower florets
- 3 cups vegetable broth
- ½ cup full-fat coconut milk
- Salt and pepper to taste

Instructions:

1. Heat oil in a large pot. Add onion and sauté until translucent.
2. Add broccoli, cauliflower, and broth. Bring to a boil, then reduce to simmer for 20 minutes.
3. Blend soup until smooth and creamy. Stir in coconut milk and season.
4. Serve warm.

Expert Tip:

For extra protein, stir in a tablespoon of hemp seeds before blending.

Cruciferous vegetables like broccoli and cauliflower may support detox pathways and contain fiber, vitamins C and K. Cooking them reduces goitrogens, making them safer for thyroid health in moderation.

Cucumber Avocado Salad with Lemon-Herb Dressing

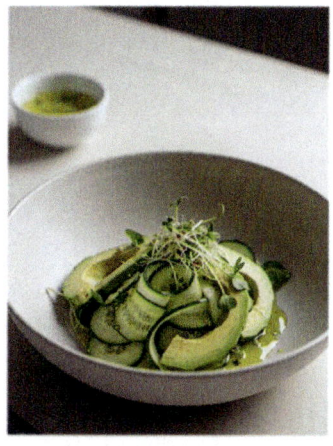

Prep Time: 10 minutes

Cook Time: None

Serving Size: 2–3 servings

Nutritional Value (per serving): Calories: 220 | Carbs: 10g | Protein: 3g | Fat: 18g | Fiber: 7g

Ingredients:

- 1 large cucumber, sliced
- 1 ripe avocado, diced
- 2 tablespoons chopped fresh dill or parsley
- Juice of 1 lemon
- 1 tablespoon extra-virgin olive oil
- Salt and pepper to taste

Instructions:

1. In a bowl, combine cucumber, avocado, and herbs.
2. Drizzle with lemon juice and olive oil. Toss gently.
3. Season to taste and serve immediately.

Expert Tip:

Add a pinch of ground flaxseed for a boost of omega-3s and fiber without altering the taste.

Hydrating and packed with healthy fats, this refreshing salad supports skin, hormonal health, and inflammation reduction—especially helpful in managing Graves' Disease symptoms.

SNACKS AND DESSERTS

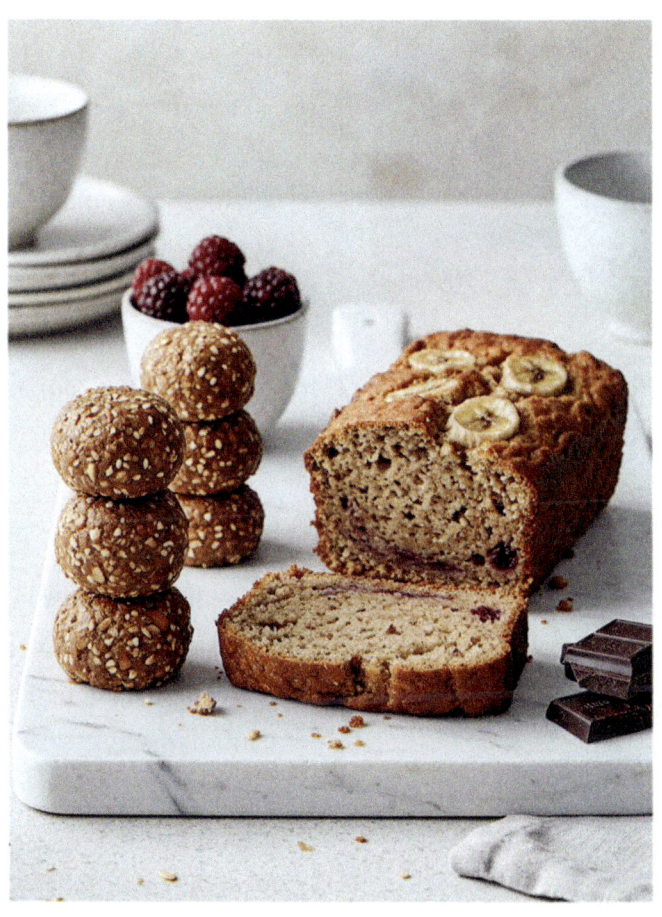

Almond Butter Energy Bites

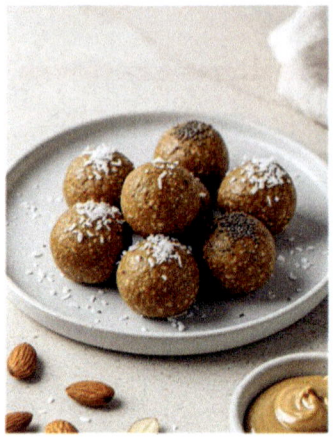

Prep Time: 10 minutes

Cook Time: None (chill for 20 minutes)

Serving Size: 12 bites

Nutritional Value (per bite):

Calories: 120 | Carbs: 10g | Protein: 4g | Fat: 7g | Fiber: 2g

Ingredients:

- 1 cup rolled oats (gluten-free if needed)
- ½ cup natural almond butter
- 2 tablespoons ground flaxseed
- 2 tablespoons chia seeds
- 2 tablespoons maple syrup or honey
- 1 teaspoon vanilla extract
- ¼ teaspoon sea salt

Instructions:

1. Mix all ingredients in a bowl until combined.
2. Roll into 1-inch balls. Chill in the refrigerator for 20–30 minutes to set.
3. Store in an airtight container in the fridge for up to 1 week.

Turmeric-Spiced Roasted Chickpeas

> *Expert Tip:*
> *Add a tablespoon of hemp seeds for extra omega-3s and protein without affecting flavor.*

> *These no-bake bites are packed with protein, fiber, and healthy fats—perfect for a quick energy boost without the crash. Almond butter supports steady blood sugar and energy, which is crucial for thyroid balance.*

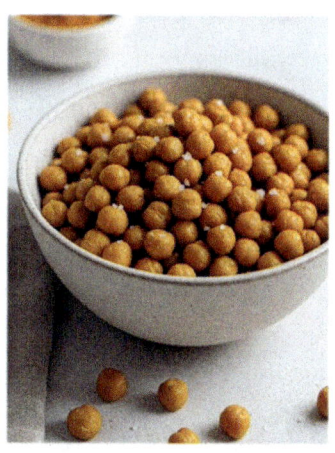

Prep Time: 5 minutes

Cook Time: 30–40 minutes

Serving Size: 4 servings

Nutritional Value (per serving):

Calories: 160 | Carbs: 18g | Protein: 6g | Fat: 6g | Fiber: 5g

Ingredients:

- 1 can chickpeas, drained and rinsed
- 1 tablespoon olive oil
- ½ teaspoon turmeric
- ½ teaspoon paprika
- ¼ teaspoon garlic powder
- ¼ teaspoon sea salt

Instructions:

1. Preheat oven to 400°F (200°C). Pat chickpeas dry with a towel.
2. Toss with oil and spices. Spread on a baking sheet in a single layer.
3. Roast for 30–40 minutes, shaking pan occasionally, until crispy.
4. Cool slightly before snacking.

Expert Tip:

For extra crunch, leave the chickpeas in the oven with the door slightly ajar for 10 minutes after roasting.

Crispy roasted chickpeas make a satisfying snack high in fiber and plant protein. Turmeric adds an anti-inflammatory kick, supporting immune and thyroid health.

Chia Pudding with Berries and Coconut Milk

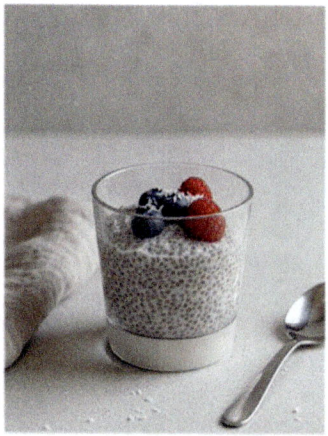

Prep Time: 5 minutes

Cook Time: None (chill overnight)

Serving Size: 2 servings

Nutritional Value (per serving):

Calories: 210 | Carbs: 14g | Protein: 5g | Fat: 15g | Fiber: 8g

Ingredients:

- ¼ cup chia seeds
- 1 cup full-fat coconut milk
- 1 teaspoon vanilla extract
- 1 tablespoon maple syrup (optional)
- ½ cup mixed berries (fresh or thawed)

Instructions:

1. In a jar or bowl, combine chia seeds, coconut milk, vanilla, and maple syrup.
2. Stir well and refrigerate overnight (or at least 4 hours).
3. Top with berries before serving.

Expert Tip:

Double the batch for a ready-made breakfast or snack that lasts several days.

Chia seeds are rich in omega-3 fatty acids, fiber, and antioxidants. This creamy pudding is naturally sweetened and supports digestion, energy, and hormonal balance.

Frozen Banana Almond Bites

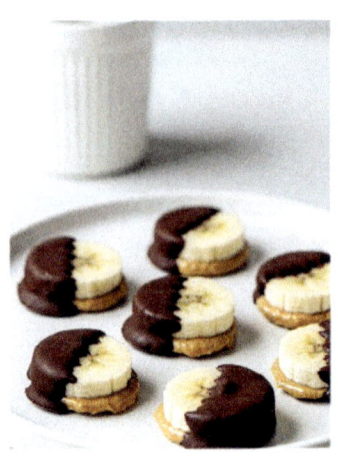

Prep Time: 10 minutes

Cook Time: Freeze for 1 hour

Serving Size: 6–8 pieces

Nutritional Value (per serving):

Calories: 100 | Carbs: 13g | Protein: 2g | Fat: 5g | Fiber: 2g

Ingredients:

- 1 ripe banana
- 2 tablespoons almond butter
- 1 tablespoon dark chocolate chips (optional)
- 1 tablespoon chopped walnuts

Instructions:

1. Slice banana into ½-inch rounds and top half with almond butter.
2. Sandwich with remaining banana slices.
3. Top with chocolate chips and walnuts if using. Freeze on a lined tray for 1 hour.
4. Enjoy frozen or slightly thawed.

Expert Tip:

Choose dark chocolate chips (70%+) for antioxidant benefits and lower sugar content.

These creamy frozen treats are naturally sweet, dairy-free, and rich in potassium—great for adrenal and thyroid support. They feel indulgent but are actually guilt-free.

Baked Apple Slices with Cinnamon and Coconut

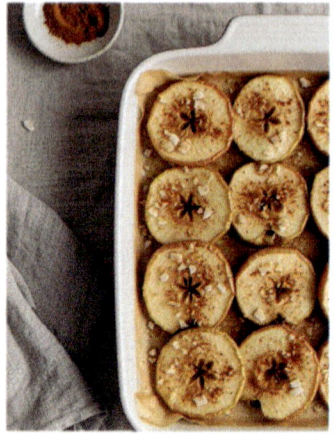

Prep Time: 5 minutes

Cook Time: 20 minutes

Serving Size: 2 servings

Nutritional Value (per serving):

Calories: 130 | Carbs: 20g | Protein: 1g | Fat: 5g | Fiber: 4g

Ingredients:

- 1 large apple, thinly sliced
- 1 tablespoon coconut oil
- ½ teaspoon ground cinnamon
- 1 tablespoon unsweetened shredded coconut

Instructions:

1. Preheat oven to 375°F (190°C).
2. Toss apple slices with coconut oil and cinnamon. Spread on a baking dish.
3. Bake for 20 minutes, until tender.
4. Sprinkle with shredded coconut before serving.

Expert Tip:

Add a few chopped walnuts or pecans for extra crunch and selenium.

Warm cinnamon apples are naturally sweet, calming, and supportive of blood sugar regulation. This dessert is comfort food at its healthiest.

Pumpkin Seed Trail Mix

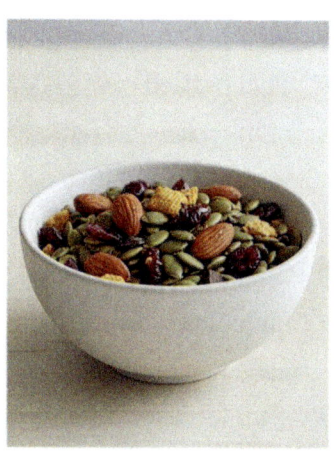

Prep Time: 5 minutes

Cook Time: None

Serving Size: 6 servings

Nutritional Value (per serving):

Calories: 180 | Carbs: 12g | Protein: 6g | Fat: 12g | Fiber: 3g

Ingredients:

- ½ cup raw pumpkin seeds
- ¼ cup almonds
- ¼ cup walnuts
- ¼ cup dried cranberries (unsweetened if possible)
- 2 tablespoons dark chocolate chips (70% cacao or higher)
- 1 tablespoon shredded coconut

Instructions:

1. Mix all ingredients in a bowl.
2. Store in an airtight container at room temperature for up to a week.

a flavorful twist without added sugar.

Pumpkin seeds are a powerhouse of zinc and magnesium—both crucial for thyroid hormone production and immune health. This trail mix is great for on-the-go snacking with a balanced blend of nutrients.

Expert Tip:

Add a pinch of sea salt or a sprinkle of cinnamon for

Avocado Cocoa Mousse

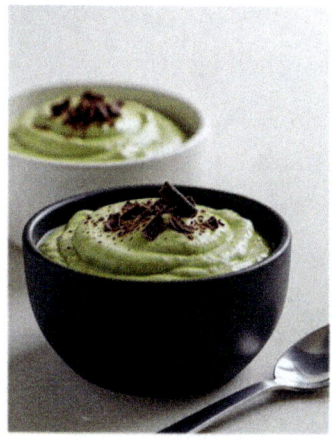

Prep Time: 10 minutes

Cook Time: None

Serving Size: 2 servings

Nutritional Value (per serving):

Calories: 220 | Carbs: 15g | Protein: 3g | Fat: 18g | Fiber: 6g

Ingredients:

- 1 ripe avocado
- 2 tablespoons raw cacao powder
- 2 tablespoons maple syrup
- 1 teaspoon vanilla extract
- 1 tablespoon almond milk (to thin, optional)

Instructions:

1. Blend all ingredients in a food processor or blender until smooth and creamy.
2. Add almond milk as needed for desired texture.
3. Chill for 20 minutes and serve with fresh berries or coconut flakes.

Expert Tip:

Use cacao instead of cocoa powder for a richer antioxidant profile and better thyroid support.

This creamy, decadent dessert is loaded with heart-healthy fats and antioxidants from avocado and cocoa. It's a smart, anti-inflammatory alternative to sugary puddings.

Carrot Cake Bliss Balls

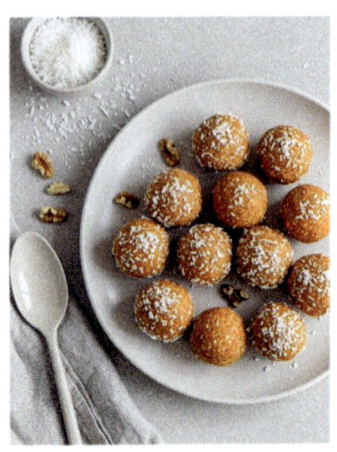

Prep Time: 15 minutes

Cook Time: None

Serving Size: 10 balls

Nutritional Value (per ball):

Calories: 90 | Carbs: 10g | Protein: 2g | Fat: 5g | Fiber: 2g

Ingredients:

- 1 cup grated carrot
- ½ cup oats
- ½ cup pitted Medjool dates
- ¼ cup walnuts
- 1 tablespoon chia seeds
- ½ teaspoon cinnamon
- ⅛ teaspoon nutmeg

Instructions:

1. Pulse all ingredients in a food processor until a sticky dough forms.
2. Roll into bite-sized balls. Refrigerate for 30 minutes before eating.
3. Store in fridge for up to 5 days.

Expert Tip:

Roll in shredded coconut or crushed nuts for a pretty finish and added texture.

Carrots are rich in beta-carotene and fiber, and these bliss balls are sweetened naturally with dates and spiced with warming cinnamon and nutmeg.

Baked Pears with Walnuts and Cinnamon

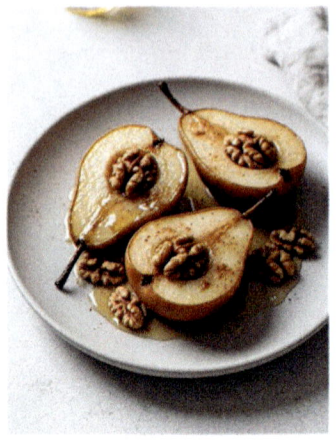

Prep Time: 5 minutes

Cook Time: 25 minutes

Serving Size: 2 servings

Nutritional Value (per serving):

Calories: 160 | Carbs: 22g | Protein: 2g | Fat: 7g | Fiber: 4g

Ingredients:

- 1 ripe pear, halved and cored
- 2 teaspoons coconut oil
- 2 tablespoons chopped walnuts
- ½ teaspoon ground cinnamon
- 1 teaspoon maple syrup (optional)

Instructions:

1. Preheat oven to 375°F (190°C).
2. Place pear halves in a baking dish. Drizzle with coconut oil and sprinkle with walnuts and cinnamon.
3. Bake for 20–25 minutes until soft and fragrant.
4. Drizzle with maple syrup before serving, if desired.

Golden Milk Bites

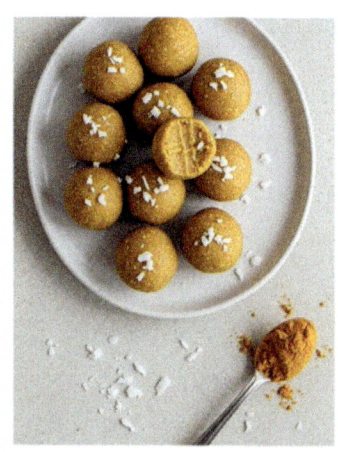

Expert Tip:

For a dairy-free creamy topping, add a dollop of unsweetened coconut yogurt or cashew cream.

Pears are high in fiber and gentle on digestion. When baked with cinnamon and walnuts, they create a simple, thyroid-friendly dessert that feels indulgent but supports wellness.

Prep Time: 10 minutes

Cook Time: None

Serving Size: 10 bites

Nutritional Value (per bite):

Calories: 100 | Carbs: 9g | Protein: 2g | Fat: 6g | Fiber: 2g

Ingredients:

➢ ½ cup pitted dates

- ½ cup almond flour
- ¼ cup unsweetened shredded coconut
- 1 tablespoon coconut oil
- 1 teaspoon turmeric
- ½ teaspoon cinnamon
- Pinch of black pepper (boosts curcumin absorption)

Instructions:

1. Blend all ingredients in a food processor until mixture sticks together.
2. Roll into small balls. Refrigerate 30 minutes before serving.
3. Store in an airtight container in the fridge for up to 1 week.

Expert Tip:

Add a tiny piece of fresh ginger or a pinch of ground ginger for an extra zing and digestive boost.

Inspired by anti-inflammatory golden milk, these bites combine turmeric, coconut, and dates to offer a warming, nourishing snack with a touch of natural sweetness.

Sweet Potato & Tahini Cookies

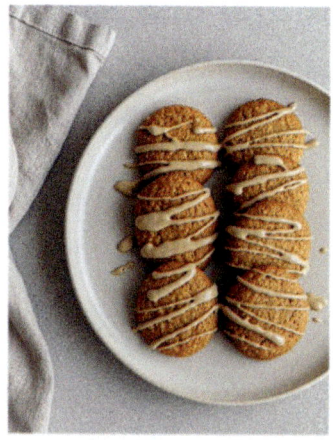

Prep Time: 10 minutes

Cook Time: 20 minutes

Serving Size: 10 cookies

Nutritional Value (per cookie):

Calories: 110 | Carbs: 12g | Protein: 2g | Fat: 6g | Fiber: 2g

Ingredients:

- ½ cup mashed cooked sweet potato
- ¼ cup tahini
- 2 tablespoons maple syrup
- 1 teaspoon vanilla extract
- ½ teaspoon cinnamon
- ½ teaspoon baking soda
- ¾ cup almond flour

Instructions:

1. Preheat oven to 350°F (175°C) and line a baking sheet with parchment paper.
2. In a bowl, mix mashed sweet potato, tahini, maple syrup, and vanilla.
3. Add cinnamon, baking soda, and almond flour. Stir until a dough forms.

4. Scoop dough into small balls, flatten slightly, and place on the baking sheet.
5. Bake for 18–20 minutes, then cool before serving.

Expert Tip:

Add chopped walnuts or dark chocolate chips for a nutrient-dense twist.

Sweet potatoes are rich in beta-carotene; a key antioxidant that helps reduce inflammation and support thyroid function. These cookies are soft, subtly sweet, and free of refined sugar and gluten.

Coconut Yogurt Parfait with Berries and Seeds

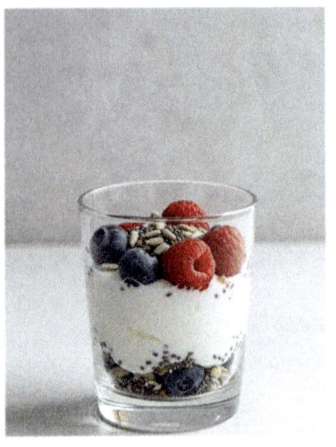

Prep Time: 5 minutes

Cook Time: None

Serving Size: 2 parfaits

Nutritional Value (per serving):

Calories: 180 | Carbs: 15g | Protein: 4g | Fat: 12g | Fiber: 5g

Ingredients:

- 1 cup unsweetened coconut yogurt
- ½ cup mixed berries (blueberries, raspberries, strawberries)
- 1 tablespoon chia seeds
- 1 tablespoon pumpkin seeds
- 1 tablespoon hemp seeds
- 1 teaspoon honey or maple syrup (optional)

Expert Tip:

Make it a meal by adding ¼ cup of gluten-free granola for extra crunch and fiber.

This parfait is a refreshing, probiotic-rich snack or dessert that supports gut health and hormone balance. It's naturally sweet and packed with antioxidants.

Instructions:

1. In a glass or jar, layer coconut yogurt, berries, and seeds.
2. Drizzle with a touch of honey or maple syrup if desired.
3. Enjoy immediately or chill for later.

Spiced Quinoa Pudding

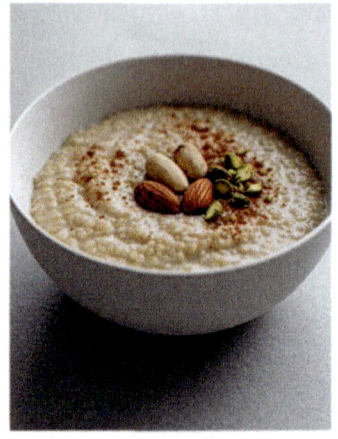

Prep Time: 5 minutes

Cook Time: 20 minutes

Serving Size: 2 servings

Nutritional Value (per serving):

Calories: 220 | Carbs: 30g | Protein: 6g | Fat: 8g | Fiber: 4g

Ingredients:

- ½ cup cooked quinoa
- 1 cup almond milk (or coconut milk)
- 1 tablespoon maple syrup
- ½ teaspoon cinnamon
- ⅛ teaspoon nutmeg
- ½ teaspoon vanilla extract
- Pinch of sea salt

Instructions:

1. In a saucepan, combine all ingredients and bring to a simmer over medium heat.
2. Cook, stirring occasionally, for 15–20 minutes until thick and creamy.
3. Serve warm, topped with berries or chopped nuts.

Expert Tip:

Store leftovers in the fridge and reheat with a splash of milk for a quick, cozy snack.

A warming, creamy alternative to traditional rice pudding, this version uses quinoa—a complete plant protein—and thyroid-supportive spices like cinnamon and nutmeg.

Cucumber & Hummus Bites

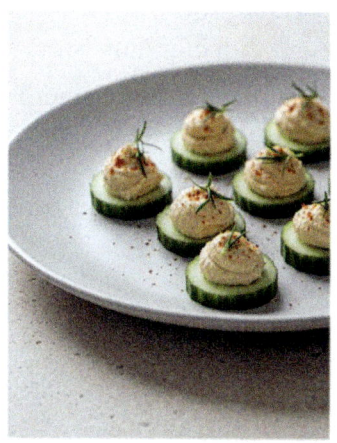

Prep Time: 5 minutes

Cook Time: None

Serving Size: 1 (makes about 8 bites)

Nutritional Value (per serving):

Calories: 100 | Carbs: 8g | Protein: 3g | Fat: 6g | Fiber: 3g

Ingredients:

- ½ cucumber, sliced into rounds
- ¼ cup hummus (store-bought or homemade)
- Paprika or sesame seeds (optional garnish)

Instructions:

1. Spread 1 teaspoon of hummus on each cucumber slice.
2. Sprinkle with paprika or sesame seeds for added flavor.
3. Serve immediately as a cooling, protein-rich snack.

Expert Tip:

Add a slice of avocado or roasted red pepper on top for extra flavor and healthy fats.

Sometimes the simplest snacks are the most satisfying. These crunchy cucumber bites topped with creamy hummus offer fiber, protein, and a refreshing way to stabilize blood sugar between meals.

No-Bake Fig & Nut Bars

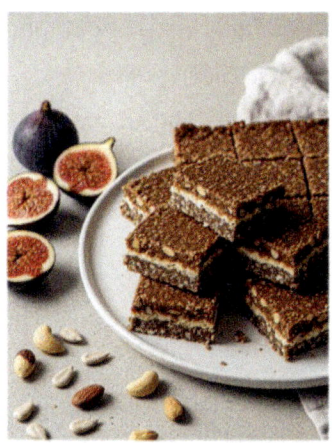

Prep Time: 10 minutes

Cook Time: Chill for 30 minutes

Serving Size: 8 small bars

Nutritional Value (per bar):

Calories: 160 | Carbs: 14g | Protein: 4g | Fat: 10g | Fiber: 3g

Ingredients:

- ½ cup dried figs (stems removed)
- ½ cup raw almonds
- ½ cup walnuts
- 1 tablespoon chia seeds
- 1 tablespoon coconut oil
- Pinch of cinnamon
- Pinch of sea salt

Instructions:

1. Pulse all ingredients in a food processor until mixture is sticky and holds together.
2. Press into a parchment-lined dish and chill for 30 minutes.
3. Slice into bars and store in the fridge for up to a week.

Expert Tip:

Soak the figs in warm water for 10 minutes before blending if they're a bit dry.

Figs provide natural sweetness and fiber, while mixed nuts offer healthy fats and minerals like magnesium and zinc. These bars are perfect for a quick energy boost without processed ingredients.

BONUS

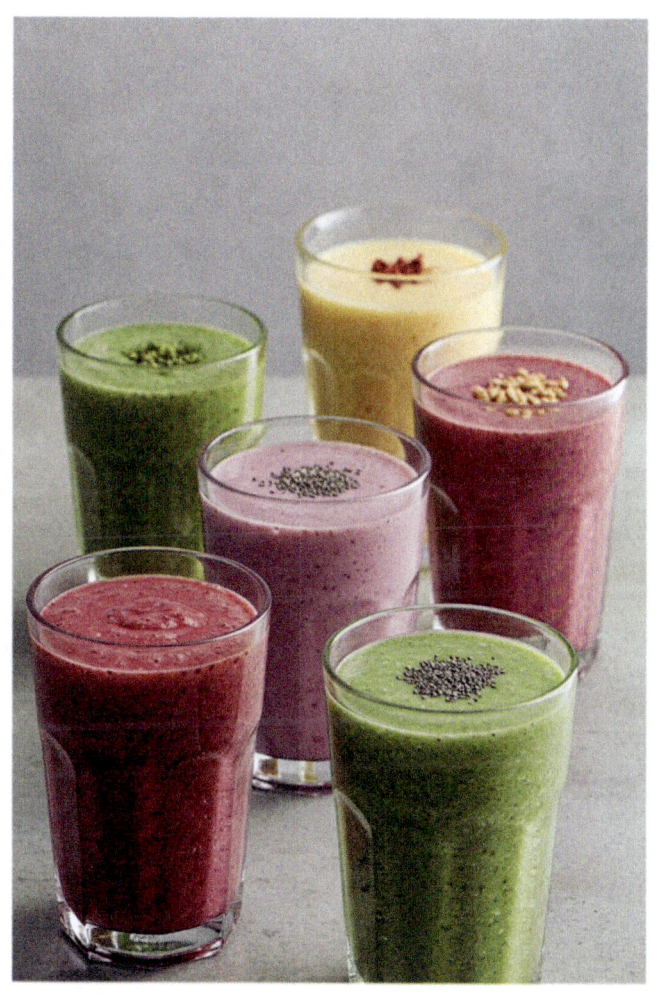

Berry Brazil Nut Boost Smoothie

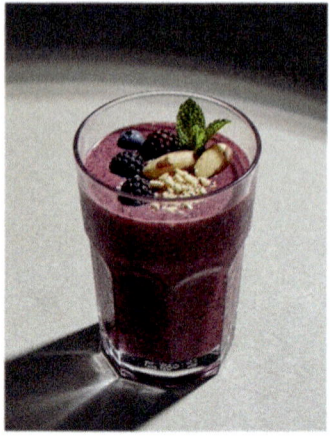

Prep Time: 5 minutes

Cooking Time: None

Servings: 1

Nutritional Value:

Rich in selenium, antioxidants, healthy fats, and fiber.

Ingredients:

- 1 cup frozen mixed berries (blueberries, raspberries, strawberries)
- 1 cup unsweetened almond milk
- 2 Brazil nuts
- 1 tablespoon chia seeds
- ½ banana
- 1 teaspoon maple syrup (optional)

Instructions:

1. Add all ingredients to a blender.
2. Blend on high until smooth and creamy.
3. Pour into a glass and enjoy immediately.

Expert Tip:

Limit Brazil nuts to 2–3 per serving to avoid excessive selenium, which can impact thyroid function when consumed in large quantities.

Brazil nuts are one of the richest natural sources of selenium, a mineral crucial for thyroid hormone production and antioxidant defense. Pairing them with berries amps up the anti-inflammatory benefits.

Golden Pineapple Turmeric Smoothie

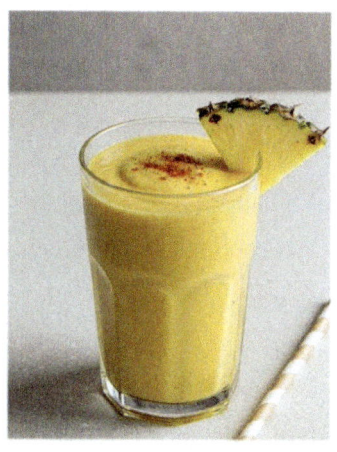

Prep Time: 5 minutes

Cooking Time: None

Servings: 1

Nutritional Value:

Anti-inflammatory, rich in vitamin C and digestive enzymes.

Ingredients:

- 1 cup frozen pineapple
- ½ teaspoon ground turmeric
- 1 teaspoon grated fresh ginger
- ¾ cup unsweetened coconut milk
- ½ frozen banana
- Dash of black pepper (enhances turmeric absorption)

> *Turmeric's active compound, curcumin, offers powerful anti-inflammatory benefits—ideal for autoimmune thyroid support.*

Instructions:

1. Add all ingredients to a blender and blend until smooth.
2. Taste and add more ginger or turmeric if desired.
3. Serve immediately.

Expert Tip:

Black pepper boosts curcumin absorption by up to 2000%—don't skip it

Green Zinc Detox Smoothie

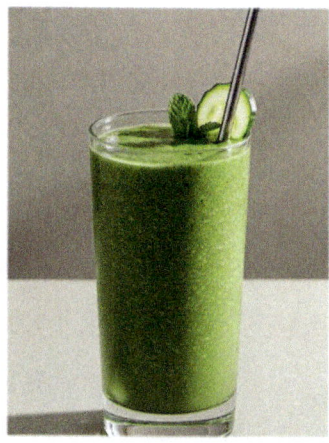

Prep Time: 5 minutes

Cooking Time: None

Servings: 1

Nutritional Value:

Rich in zinc, antioxidants, hydration, and fiber.

Ingredients:

- 1 cup fresh spinach
- ½ cucumber, peeled and sliced
- Juice of ½ lemon
- 1 tablespoon pumpkin seeds
- ½ avocado
- 1 cup coconut water
- 1 teaspoon honey (optional)

Instructions:

1. Blend all ingredients until creamy and smooth.
2. Taste and adjust with honey or lemon as needed.
3. Pour into a glass and enjoy chilled.

Expert Tip:

To increase detox support, add a few fresh parsley leaves—an excellent natural cleanser.

This mineral-rich smoothie combines zinc-packed spinach and pumpkin seeds with hydrating cucumber and detoxifying lemon for thyroid and immune support.

Coconut Blueberry Protein Smoothie

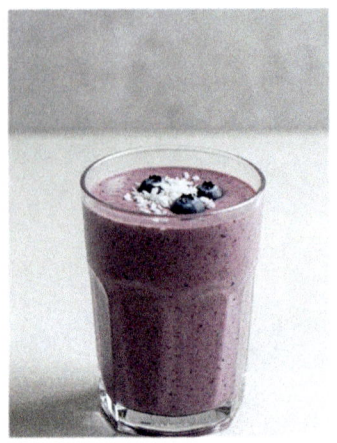

Prep Time: 5 minutes

Cooking Time: None

Servings: 1

Nutritional Value:

Rich in protein, omega-3s, antioxidants, and healthy fats.

Ingredients:

- 1 cup frozen blueberries
- 1 scoop unflavored collagen or clean protein powder
- 1 tablespoon chia seeds
- 1 cup full-fat coconut milk
- ½ teaspoon cinnamon

This creamy, protein-rich smoothie is great for post-workout recovery or a filling breakfast. Coconut milk provides healthy fats, while blueberries and chia fight inflammation.

Instructions:

1. Blend all ingredients together until smooth.
2. Let sit for 2 minutes to allow chia to thicken.
3. Serve with a sprinkle of cinnamon on top.

Expert Tip:

Add ½ zucchini (peeled and frozen) to increase volume and fiber without altering taste.

Papaya Ginger Digestion Smoothie

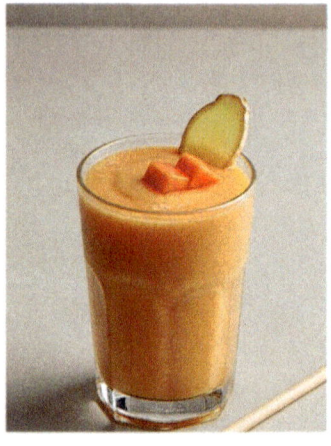

Prep Time: 5 minutes

Cooking Time: None

Servings: 1

Nutritional Value:

Great source of enzymes, vitamin C, and anti-inflammatory compounds.

Ingredients:

- 1 cup fresh or frozen papaya
- 1 teaspoon grated fresh ginger
- Juice of ½ lime
- 1 tablespoon ground flaxseed
- ¾ cup coconut water
- Handful of ice

Instructions:

1. Add all ingredients to a blender.
2. Blend on high until silky smooth.
3. Enjoy cold, especially after meals.

Expert Tip:

Fresh papaya works best, but frozen is fine—just make sure it's ripe for optimal enzyme activity.

Papaya is rich in enzymes that aid digestion and reduce inflammation. Combined with gut-friendly ginger, this smoothie helps calm the digestive tract and support thyroid health.

Cinnamon Apple Pie Smoothie

Prep Time: 5 minutes

Cooking Time: None

Servings: 1

Nutritional Value:

High in fiber, vitamin C, and natural anti-inflammatory compounds.

Ingredients:

- 1 medium apple (peeled and chopped)
- ½ banana
- 1 tablespoon almond butter
- ½ teaspoon cinnamon
- ¾ cup unsweetened oat milk
- Handful of ice

Instructions:

1. Combine all ingredients in a blender.
2. Blend until creamy and smooth.
3. Sprinkle with extra cinnamon before serving if desired.

Expert Tip:

For extra protein, add a tablespoon of hemp seeds or a scoop of clean protein powder.

Strawberry Basil Calm Smoothie

All the cozy flavors of apple pie without the sugar crash! This smoothie stabilizes blood sugar and supports metabolism with cinnamon and fiber-rich apples.

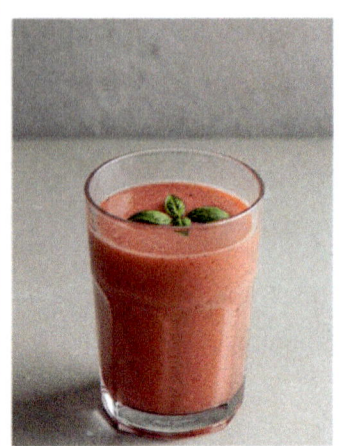

Prep Time: 5 minutes

Cooking Time: None

Servings: 1

Nutritional Value:

Vitamin C, antioxidants, stress-regulating compounds.

Ingredients:

- ➢ 1 cup frozen strawberries
- ➢ 4–5 fresh basil leaves
- ➢ ½ cup plain unsweetened yogurt (dairy-free if needed)
- ➢ ½ cup almond milk
- ➢ 1 teaspoon flaxseed
- ➢ Optional: ½ teaspoon honey

> *Basil has adaptogenic properties that may help regulate stress—a major trigger for thyroid flares. Paired with vitamin C-rich strawberries, this is a refreshing and calming blend.*

Instructions:

1. Blend all ingredients until smooth and creamy.
2. Taste and add honey if desired.
3. Pour into a chilled glass and enjoy.

Expert Tip:

For an extra cooling effect in summer, blend in a few ice cubes and top with a basil leaf.

Pineapple Turmeric Anti-Inflammatory Smoothie

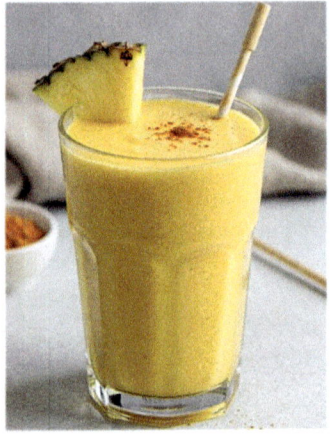

Prep Time: 5 minutes

Cook Time: None

Serving Size: 1

Nutritional Value:

Approx. 220 calories, 4g protein, 7g fat, 38g carbs, rich in vitamin C, manganese, and curcumin

Ingredients:

- 1 cup fresh or frozen pineapple chunks
- 1 banana
- 1/2 tsp ground turmeric
- 1/2-inch piece of fresh ginger (or 1/4 tsp ground ginger)
- 1 tbsp flaxseed meal
- 1/2 cup unsweetened coconut milk
- 1/2 cup water or more as needed
- Juice of 1/2 a lemon
- A pinch of black pepper (to enhance turmeric absorption)

Instructions:

1. Add all ingredients to a blender.
2. Blend on high until smooth.

3. Add more water to adjust consistency if needed.
4. Serve immediately.

Expert Tip:

Always pair turmeric with black pepper and a healthy fat like flaxseed for optimal absorption of curcumin, its active compound.

Turmeric is a powerful anti-inflammatory spice that may help reduce symptoms associated with autoimmune conditions like Graves' disease.

Creamy Spinach & Pear Green Smoothie

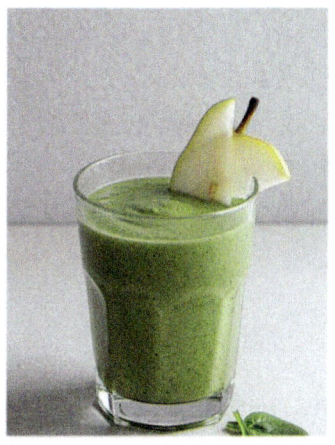

Prep Time: 5 minutes

Cook Time: None

Serving Size: 1

Nutritional Value:

Approx. 180 calories, 3g protein, 4g fat, 36g carbs, high in vitamin K and fiber

Ingredients:

- 1 ripe pear, cored and sliced
- 1 cup fresh spinach
- 1/2 banana
- 1/4 avocado
- 1 tbsp chia seeds
- 1/2 cup unsweetened almond milk
- 1/2 cup water or ice

Instructions:

1. Combine all ingredients in a blender.
2. Blend until smooth and creamy.
3. Pour into a glass and enjoy fresh.

Expert Tip:

Soaking chia seeds for a few minutes before blending can make the smoothie easier to digest and even creamier.

Spinach is a rich source of magnesium and iron—minerals often depleted in those with thyroid imbalances.

Zinc-Rich Chocolate Pumpkin Smoothie

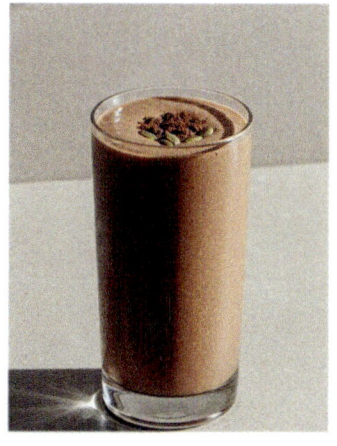

Prep Time: 5 minutes

Cook Time: None

Serving Size: 1

Nutritional Value:

Approx. 250 calories, 8g protein, 10g fat, 28g carbs, high in zinc, iron, and fiber

Ingredients:

- 1/2 cup pure pumpkin purée (unsweetened)
- 1 frozen banana
- 1 tbsp raw cacao powder
- 2 tbsp pumpkin seeds
- 1 cup unsweetened oat milk
- 1/2 tsp cinnamon
- 1/4 tsp vanilla extract
- Ice cubes as needed

Instructions:

1. Blend all ingredients until smooth.
2. Add more milk or ice for desired texture.
3. Serve cold.

Expert Tip:

Roasting pumpkin seeds before blending can

enhance flavor, but use raw for maximum nutrient preservation.

Pumpkin seeds and cocoa are great plant-based sources of zinc, a vital mineral for thyroid hormone production.

CONCLUSION

If you've made it this far—thank you. Truly. Writing this book has been a labor of love, and knowing you're holding it in your hands, cooking from its pages, and taking steps toward healing your thyroid means everything.

Living with Graves' disease isn't always easy. It can feel confusing, overwhelming, and isolating at times. But I hope this book has shown you that with the right tools, knowledge, and nourishing meals, you can begin to take back your power—one bite at a time.

These recipes weren't just created to fill your plate—they were carefully designed to support your thyroid, calm inflammation, and make you feel more like you again. I wanted every smoothie, every main dish, and every little snack to be more than just healthy—I wanted them to be satisfying, flavorful, and easy to love. Because food should be joyful, not stressful. Healing should feel empowering, not limiting.

Remember, you don't need to do everything perfectly. Progress is so much more important than perfection. Maybe you start with one new recipe a week. Maybe you just begin by adding more whole foods to your grocery cart. Wherever you are in your journey, know that even the smallest steps forward matter.

You've already done something powerful by choosing to understand your body and nourish it intentionally. That's a beautiful act of self-care—and one that deserves to be celebrated.

My wish is that this book becomes a trusted guide in your kitchen and a comforting friend on your journey. I hope it gives you hope on the hard days, and energy on the good ones. And most of all, I hope it helps you reconnect with the vibrant, capable, strong version of yourself—the one that Graves' disease doesn't define.

Stay curious. Stay kind to yourself. Keep listening to your body. And above all, don't forget how far you've come.

Wishing you a nourished, balanced, and thriving future.

With warmth and gratitude,

Thalia Rowen

ABOUT THE AUTHOR

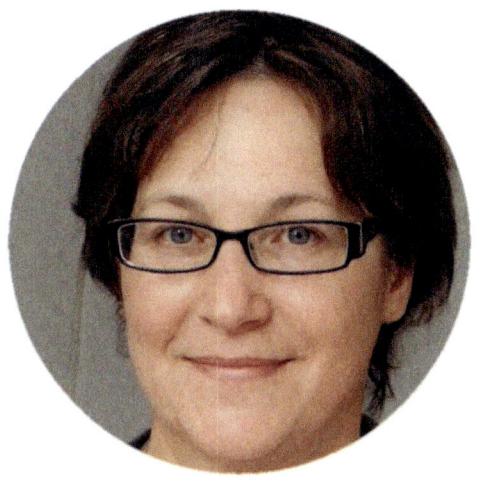

Thalia Rowen is a health-focused cookbook author with a deep passion for creating nourishing, delicious meals that support well-being without sacrificing flavor. With a background in holistic nutrition and a love for simple, whole-food ingredients, Thalia is dedicated to helping others feel their best—one recipe at a time.

Her cookbooks are crafted with care to be approachable, inspiring, and rooted in real-life needs, especially for those navigating specific health conditions. Whether you're just beginning your wellness journey or looking to deepen your relationship with food, Thalia's recipes are designed to empower you in the kitchen and support a vibrant, balanced life.

When she's not developing new recipes, Thalia enjoys mindful cooking, long nature walks, and sharing wholesome meals with her loved ones.

Printed in Dunstable, United Kingdom